Foreword by Amy Weintraub,
author of *Yoga for Depression*

JENNIE LEE

true yoga

PRACTICING *with the* YOGA SUTRAS
for HAPPINESS & SPIRITUAL
FULFILLMENT

Llewellyn Worldwide
Woodbury, Minnesota

FIRST EDITION
First Printing, 2016

Book design by Bob Gaul
Cover art by iStockphoto.com/34298342/©CPD-Lab
            iStockphoto.com/1910736/©molotovcoketail
Cover design by Ellen Lawson
Editing by Ed Day
Part Page art by iStockphoto.com/34298342/©CPD-Lab
            iStockphoto.com/1910736/©molotovcoketail

Llewellyn Publications is a registered trademark of Llewellyn Worldwide Ltd.

Library of Congress Cataloging-in-Publication Data (Pending)
ISBN: 978-0-7387-4625-8

Llewellyn Publications
A Division of Llewellyn Worldwide Ltd.
2143 Wooddale Drive
Woodbury, MN 55125-2989
www.llewellyn.com

Printed in the United States of America

Disclaimer

The material in this book is not intended as a substitute for trained medical or psychological advice. Readers are advised to consult their personal healthcare professionals regarding treatment. The publisher and the author assume no liability for any injuries caused to the reader that may result from the reader's use of the content contained herein and recommend common sense when contemplating the practices described in the work.

Contents

Foreword

Over the centuries, many have studied and made commentary on the Yoga Sutras of Patanjali. Being unfamiliar with Jennie Lee as a teacher, when I received *True Yoga: Practicing with the Yoga Sutras for Happiness and Spiritual Fulfillment,* I questioned what she might have to offer that was new. What I found was a teacher who recognized her Self in the classical text, as though already knowing it by heart. Her interpretive commentary is grounded in five different translations, but comes from direct reflection on their meaning in her life. Jennie Lee engages with the Yoga Sutras as one who lives them, and she shares from the perspective that learning is an affirmation of lived experience, not memorization. As such, she gives us this gift—a beautifully written translation and commentary rooted in compassion, in which we too can see ourselves reflected. This way of connecting with the Yoga Sutras—through personal and direct communication, where the reader can have that "ah-ha" moment of recognition—is the most valuable way to learn.

In one of my favorite commentaries on the Sutras, Swami Venkatesananda makes the distinction between "conveying" and "communication." One can convey information, but meaning comes from true communication. "In communication," he says, "misunderstanding does not take place, because in communication the two become one. They are on the same wavelength and the meaning is transmitted from heart-to-heart." [1] This kind of communication does not come easily through words alone. And yet, it can happen when we find a text that so meets us, heart-to-heart, that we immediately understand its meaning. This is the way the Yoga Sutras are meant to be studied. The commentary you hold in your hands may be such a vehicle for this heart-to-heart connection between you and the deeper meaning of the Sutras.

Related to each Sutra, you will find daily practices, self-inquiry questions, and affirmations that help you not only to integrate the wisdom of the Sutras in your life but will also bring you more joy. Rather than the discipline emphasized in some Yoga Sutra commentaries, the viewpoint this one invites you to hold is that of a growing Self-awareness combined with compassion for who you truly are beneath mood and story and

---

1   Swami Venkatesananda, *The Yoga Sutras of Patanjali with Commentary*, 3rd rev. ed. (Delhi: MB, 2008).

the challenges you face in daily life. This is a commentary that speaks directly, heart to heart. Just listen and respond.

—Amy Weintraub, founder of the
LifeForce Yoga Healing Institute and author of
Yoga for Depression and *Yoga Skills for Therapists*

This book is dedicated to God,
the greatest Love of all.

Introduction

Right now... are you happy? If things are going well, you probably are. If not, you may be feeling low. What if, no matter what was happening in your life, good or bad, you could answer, "Yes! I am happy!"

To find happiness we usually look outward to people, places, and things that bring us fulfillment. But these pleasures are often short-lived and unpredictable, so our quest renews day after day. At a certain point, whether through cynicism or suffering, we realize that external pleasures, however great, do not bring enduring gratification. And regardless of whether we have had an abundance of success or a lack thereof, while we are wasting time in our attempts to secure happiness in the world, life is ebbing away.

1

We are overdue to experience more than just ephemeral hits of happiness. The good news is, there is a way to feel purpose, meaning, and joy every day, no matter what life brings. A time-tested guide for our personal development of these experiences was given to us in the Yoga Sutras, a comprehensive list of one hundred ninety-six life-expanding teachings compiled over two thousand years ago by a sage named Patanjali. In the Sutras, we find a section referred to as the Eight Limbs of Yoga, a succinct outline of spiritual wisdom integrated with tangible practices showing us how to live life in a state of *consistent happiness*. The purpose of *True Yoga* is to illustrate how these specific Sutras can be used to claim deep, lasting joy and fulfillment, far greater than anything the external world has to offer.

My Story

Pain is a strong motivator. Although it does not have to be, pain is often the nudge we need to look beyond the temporary pleasures of life and find some new perspective. Sad but true, humans rarely leave their comfort zone unless shaken from it.

Sixteen years ago, I got the big nudge. In a painful low point, I was challenged by a rocky marriage, exhausted from a colicky baby, and frightened as I prepared for a cross-country move away from my friends, family, career, and all things familiar. I had used up my inner resources for getting back into balance and as tempting as eating, drinking, shopping, or avoiding it all in some other unhealthy way was, I knew that none of the above would take me to any kind of true fulfillment. So I started seeking a method to attain inner peace and love that would be permanent.

Coincidentally, at this same time, I was studying for a master's degree in spiritual psychology. To complete my first year, I had to write a personal theory of counseling, so I decided to use the assignment to imagine my own map to the happiness I was craving. I called it Joy Therapy and it began like this:

"Inside each of us is the radiant light of Joy. It is the Divine spark, ignited at our birth. By individual realization of our connection to the Divine Source, we find our true inner joy and our light shines forth."

Sounds kind of like one of the first Yoga Sutras, in which it is written, "United in the heart, consciousness is steadied. Then we abide in our true nature—joy." [2]

The crazy thing is that I *had not studied* the Yoga Sutras at that time! When I wrote my thesis on Joy Therapy, I was practicing only the physical aspect of yoga and had no idea that I had created a parallel model to the ancient outline for happiness outlined in the Sutras. When I discovered the full teachings of true yoga and how the headstands and downward dogs I loved were connected to this amazing science of happiness, it made perfect sense to merge my Joy Therapy into Yoga Therapy. Since then I have made Yoga Therapy my profession and shared the life-changing principles of the Sutras with hundreds of clients.

The point of the story here, however, is to illustrate that because I was truly seeking happiness at a soul level, my individual

---

2   Nischala Joy Devi, *The Secret Power of Yoga* (New York: Three Rivers Press, 2007), 18.

awareness tapped into the all-pervading Creative Consciousness and received the necessary understanding. This is the very essence of the journey the Yoga Sutras lead us in taking, to move beyond our perspective of separate, fearful individual experience to the blissful union with Divine Consciousness in which all is possible, joyful, and secure.

Many years have passed since then and life has delivered plenty of challenges for me to test what it takes to live these teachings personally, including a year of severe depression, the loss of a child and a parent, a divorce, additional cross-country moves, a decade of single parenting, and a lot of financial hardship. But through daily practice of the principles outlined here, I now experience less stress in times of trial and feel more grounded in unshakeable peace and joy. This is the reason I wrote *True Yoga*. Through this guidebook, it is my intention to show you how to have *lasting* happiness and spiritual fulfillment—no matter what challenges life throws your way.

To be truly happy is to be successful at life and, like anything worth accomplishing, these practices require dedication. We must *choose* a peaceful response in times of conflict. We must *choose* a grateful thought when we feel negative and down. We must *choose* to tell the truth even when it is not convenient. These are not always easy choices, but if we are ready to claim true happiness and security that can sustain us through all the ups and downs of life, then these choices become a small price for the serenity, power, and wisdom they bring.

For anyone interested in being happy and anyone interested in practicing true yoga, the Eight Limbs outlined in the Yoga Sutras are *essential* for success. They lead us to ease, harmony, and satisfaction in all that we undertake on a daily basis. And they illumine a concise system that opens the path to joy and connection with our own Divinity. Now, to contextualize the Eight Limbs, let us look into a brief history of the Yoga Sutras.

How the Yoga Sutras Came About

Many earlier teachings and writings contributed to the Sutras, including the *Vedas*, the *Upanishads*, Buddhist teachings, and the *Bhagavad Gita*. These were synthesized and systematized into the foundational text that is essential to our current understanding and practice of yoga, the Yoga Sutras.

Yoga Philosophy and the Vedas

The first documentation of yoga teachings dates as far back as five thousand years ago. Seals excavated from archeological sites in the Indus Valley show figures in meditative postures. Also attributed to this general time are the *Vedas*, considered the oldest religious text from which yoga philosophy comes. The word Vedas stems from the Sanskrit root word *vid*, which means "knowledge." Classical Hindu philosophy recognizes the *Vedas* as the supreme revealed scripture. It is comprised of six branches, one of which is the philosophy of yoga we are most familiar with today.

To understand how yoga fits with the rest of the Vedic teachings, a short explanation of the six branches of Hindu philosophy is helpful. Stemming from the same root word as Vedas, the first major branch is Vedanta, which translates as knowledge (*vid*) combined with *anta* meaning "end," signifying the last and highest knowledge. Vedanta is the expression of all knowledge and experience as non-dual, attesting that all things stem from One Consciousness and are part of One Reality.

Second is Sankhya philosophy, which explains how the One Consciousness appears as many things when manifested materially. The third major branch is Yoga philosophy, which delineates how we can realize our unity with the One Consciousness through specific practices that lead us from ignorance and perceived limitation to truth and liberation.

The additional three minor branches of Hindu philosophy are Mimamsa, which studies the principles of dharma or right living; Nyaya, which explores the sources of knowledge; and Vaisesika, which reduces all created expression to its basic atomic principles. Although Hindu philosophy forms the basis of the Hindu religion, they are not equivalent and should not be confused. *Yoga is not a religion.* It is a philosophy and a spiritual science. In alignment with the Vedas, Yoga philosophy acknowledges all religious truth as falling within the One Consciousness. Therefore we may hold any religious faith and blend yoga practice with our current religious customs.

The Upanishads

The ancient Vedic ceremonies were presided over by Brahmin priests who held elite status in the caste system present in India at that time. When the early yogis decided to search out direct relationship with the One Consciousness, they went into secluded natural areas to experiment with practices that could take them to a personal experience of and communion with Spirit. From this exploration came the commentaries on the *Vedas* called the *Upanishads*, which translates as "sitting down near," as in sitting near the feet of the teacher or guru.

Written approximately three thousand years ago, the *Upanishads* focus on the personal journey of spirituality. These writings teach that our true nature, which is our oneness with Spirit, can only be known experientially. The *Upanishads* introduce many of the basic themes found later in the Yoga Sutras. A mystic named Shankara is credited with writing the ten principle Upanishads, discussing themes like Karma (law of cause and effect), maya (veil of delusion, which causes the perception of duality), prana (Life Force Energy), the chakras (energy centers), mantras (sacred phrases), meditation (state of stillness in which Divine union becomes possible), and yoga sadhana (spiritual practice). These commentaries are thought to be the culmination of the *Vedas* and are exemplified by the mantra So Hum, meaning "thou art that," which recognizes the inherent Oneness of all and the need for a personal journey toward this realization.

The Bhagavad Gita

Approximately five hundred years after the Upanishads were created, Siddhartha Gautama, known as the Buddha, further expounded the need for an individual to seek ultimate understanding of truth through the scientific process of meditation. In addition, the Indian sage Vyasa crafted the epic Hindu text known as the *Mahabharata*, presenting a philosophical discourse on the four goals of life. Within the *Mahabharata* is the *Bhagavad Gita*, a metaphoric tale of yogic wisdom told through a great battle in which a young warrior named Arjuna receives counsel from Krishna on the need for selfless action, non-attachment, and other practices that enable one to place the ego in service to the soul and live in the world but not of it.

Putting It All Together: The Yoga Sutras

The most important elements of the *Vedas*, the *Upanishads*, the Buddha's teachings, and the *Bhagavad Gita* were compiled by Sri Patanjali around two thousand years ago into the text we now refer to as the Yoga Sutras. This is the key text of Raja (Royal) Yoga, which describes the complete yoga path, a scientifically organized spiritual technology for living joyfully and ultimately achieving liberation and unity consciousness.

Within the Yoga Sutras, there are four books or sections. Book One is called the Samadhipadha and discusses the advanced stages and essential nature of enlightenment—to show us the goal. Book Two is the Sadhanapadha, which outlines necessary spiritual practices to attain this liberation, as well as the obstacles we can expect along the path. It is in this book we find the essential Eight Limbs of Yoga. Book Three is the Vibhutipadha, which overviews the spiritual powers that can be expected through dedicated yoga practice. And Book Four is the Kaivalyapadha, which describes the experience of full spiritual absorption from a more philosophical standpoint.

The word *sutra* means "to string or sew," and indicates a thread of universal wisdom on which teachers would add their beads of interpretation or expansion, depending on the time, culture, and needs of their students. They were written in concise language, kept short for easier memorization. It was expected that students not intellectualize these teachings, but rather seek direct experience through reflection and personal application of the lessons.

We, too, must heed this example. Take time to contemplate and digest each one and recognize the multidimensional interpretations and applications that are possible. The Yoga Sutras are considered a living scripture, that is, a teaching that will deliver different messages depending on our level of perception. They reveal what we need at any given time for our evolution. Like a personal love letter telling us how to live better, how to avoid the pitfalls of life, these aphorisms offer non-sectarian practices and philosophical guidelines to help us experience the Divine Joy within and become free of all suffering.

The Eight Limbs of Yoga

In the second book or section of the Sutras, we find the Eight Limbs of Yoga. In Sanskrit these are called Asthaanga Yoga, *astha* meaning "eight" and *anga* meaning "intertwining limbs." They delineate external practices first and then lead into more internal, introspective ones.

True Yoga follows the order of the Eight Limbs, dividing them into three parts for clarification of how each builds on the next. Part one covers the qualities of our highest nature that we must reconnect with for inner harmony. Part two integrates actionable outer practices with inner devotion. And part three describes the deeper, more contemplative practices that take us to a blissful, unified consciousness. Eventually all are practiced simultaneously.

The stated goal of the Eight Limbs is to awaken our consciousness to its true essence beyond the stories we create about ourselves, others, and the world. As we embody these teachings personally, we achieve a clear conscience, an unprejudiced intellect, an unbreakable will, and the ability to manifest what we need when we need it, including wisdom and guidance for right decisions. Using the practices within the Eight Limbs, we become nobler, more compassionate and happier people until one day we find ourselves in joyful liberation. Our lasting happiness is measurable by the sustained inner peace we feel and our ability to remain grateful and even-minded regardless of external circumstances. Then we are true yogis.

Getting to Happiness through Willingness, Humility, and Guidance

According to yoga philosophy, enduring happiness can only come when we stop identifying with the incessant thoughts and feelings of the personality self (small s). This "I, me, mine" perspective is called the ego and it is what we normally associate with and think of as who we are. The Sutras proclaim that all of our struggles in life are because we have forgotten the truth of our being and have strayed into a belief of separation and inadequacy. Suffering will continue until we realize that our real nature is not material but spiritual and that we cannot possibly be separated from joy and peace, because they exist within our consciousness rather than in the external world.

The Sutras begin by noting that we must learn to quiet the constant fluctuations of the individual ego mind in order to experience our true Self (capital S). To realize true Self does not mean to have a deeper understanding of our individual needs, drives, desires, and dislikes, but rather it means to have the unshakeable knowledge that we are so much more than all that. We are one with the omniscience, omnipotence, and omnipresence of the Indwelling Spirit. Then we experience life through the consciousness of our soul, the unique expression of the Divine within. In this state, we function as our human selves but see from the perspective of the true Self within. Liberated from the limitations of ego consciousness, we manifest Divine Consciousness in joy and ease here and now.

To begin the journey from where we are now to this state of expanded awareness, two qualities are essential—willingness and humility. We must be willing to turn away from the common standard of pleasure-seeking and turn our humble hearts toward a greater understanding of what brings true fulfillment.

In addition, we need a guide and, although thorough, even Google does not have GPS to take us to our Divine home.

Thankfully the spiritual seekers (rishis) of India experimented with natural and spiritual laws in their quest for fulfillment. They used their own bodies and lives as the testing ground to find ways and means of achieving peace and enlightenment permanently. They systematized this information and passed along the perfect guidelines for generations to follow.

Consistency Plus Commitment Equals Success

As any traveler can attest, reading a guidebook is not enough to know a destination personally. The map is not the territory, as they say. So the next thing that is required is the effort of movement from here to there. The beauty of yoga as a spiritual science is that we need not rely upon anyone else's theories, beliefs, or reports. Metaphorically, it is time to pack our bags and board the plane. Like the saints and yogis of the past, we can seek tangible proof in the laboratories of our own bodies, minds, and souls. Everything yoga teaches can be understood by direct experience, resulting from correct and consistent practice. Only we are responsible for the creation, preservation, or destruction of our happiness.

Sadly, many will choose to be armchair travelers and stop with intellectual information. Others may orient themselves on the map but stop with just a bit of planning. Only the committed few will take the full ride and reap the results.

It takes time to comprehend the layers of meaning in each Sutra. And to succeed in achieving an expanded awareness permanently, perseverance is essential. *True Yoga* is meant to spark your interest and give you a foundation of understanding to build from as you assimilate these teachings from the inside out. The rishis gave us the keys to the kingdom, but we must unlock the gate, not by theorizing but by *applying* the practices outlined in the Eight Limbs.

Inevitably, on any journey difficulties will arise. The Sutras identify five major obstacles (Kleshas) we may encounter on our way to true happiness and liberation. All human suffering—whether it is physical, psychological, philosophical, or metaphysical—is attributed to these five Kleshas: ignorance (Avidya), ego (Asmita), attachment (Raga), aversion (Dvesa), and fear of death (Abhinivesa). Fortunately, the suffering caused by these obstacles actually serves as motivation for us to find new ways of thinking and acting in order to relieve our discomfort.

If we persevere through trials and discouragement, offering all that we are and all that we long to be in wholehearted devotion to the practices of the Eight Limbs of Yoga, we will find every need and desire satisfied. We will have personally documentable results of greater peace and joy. And we will know the Divine Self as the Yoga Sutras describe it, within and without, in form and in formlessness.

Through this unified awareness and the continued practice of true yoga in its entirety, life becomes a peaceful playground of profound joy and love. It is our Divine right to know our blissful, perfect nature and nothing can keep us from this realization if we diligently undertake the practices given for its discovery. No external pleasure will ever compare or fulfill us in the same way.

Interpreting and Using the Sutras

Because of the complex nature of most translations of the Yoga Sutras, it is difficult for the average student or even the dedicated yoga teacher to apply these teachings personally. *True Yoga*'s exploration of the Eight Limbs is not meant to be a scholarly translation, but rather a look at the practicality of the Eight Limbs of Yoga and their relevance today as guidelines for establishing harmony in both our inner and outer lives.

In order to extrapolate a consistent meaning from each Sutra, five different translations were consulted to attain a significant overview and application to modern life. The first was the classic *The Yoga Sutras of Patanjali* by Sri Swami Satchidananda, disciple of Swami Sivananda and founder of Integral Yoga Institute. He is one of the most revered Yoga masters of modern time and this translation was originally published in 1978. Second was *The Secret Power of Yoga* published in 2007 by Nischala Joy Devi, a twenty-five-year monastic student of Sri Swami Satchidananda, one of the few female translators of the Sutras. Third was *The Heart of Yoga* by T.K.V. Desikachar, son of the great yogi Sri Krishnamacharya, a well-respected publication from 1995. Fourth was *The Essence of Yoga: Reflections on the Yoga Sutras of Patanjali* by Bernard Bouanchaud, a French student of T.K.V. Desikachar published in 1997. And finally, a more obscure and esoteric look at the Sutras was included from *The Holy Science* by Sri Swami Yukteswar Giri, disciple of Mahavatar Babaji, originally published in 1949.

The following is an example of how translations differ using Sutra ii.40 to illustrate.

———————

Sri Swami Satchidananda in *The Yoga Sutras of Patanjali* translates, "By purification arises disgust for one's own body and for contact with other bodies."[3]

Nischala Joy Devi in *The Secret Power of Yoga* translates, "Through simplicity and continual refinement (Saucha), the body, thoughts, and emotions become clear reflections of the Self within."[4]

T.K.V. Desikachar in *The Heart of Yoga* translates, "When cleanliness is developed it reveals what needs to be constantly maintained and what is eternally clean. What decays is the external. What does not is deep within us."[5]

Bernard Bouanchaud in *The Essence of Yoga* translates, "Perfect mastery of the vital energy of assimilation and equilibrium brings radiance."[6]

———————

3   Sri Swami Satchidananda, *The Yoga Sutras of Patanjali* (Buckingham, VA: Integral Yoga Publications, 2012), 133.

4   Nischala Joy Devi, *The Secret Power of Yoga* (New York: Three Rivers Press, 2007), 206.

5   T.K.V. Desikachar, *The Heart of Yoga* (Rochester, VT: Inner Traditions International, 1995), 178.

6   Bernard Bouanchaud, *The Essence of Yoga* (Delhi: Indian Books Centre, 1997), 124.

Sri Swami Yukteswar Giri in *The Holy Science* does not give a specific translation of this Sutra but states more generally, "By the practice of Yama and Niyama, the eight meannesses of the human heart disappear and virtue arises."[7]

These vastly different explanations of the principle of Saucha (purity and simplicity) show how the Sutras can be confusing at first. With study and reflection one starts to find the common elements and meanings. I am not a Sanskrit scholar, therefore the interpretations given at the beginning of each chapter are not meant to be exact, literal translations of the original Sanskrit Sutra, but rather a synthesis of the five versions, offering the reader a condensed overview and study of the essential message.

For these ancient yoga teachings to be relevant to our lives today, we must see how every aspect is applicable to our needs, as well as how it leads us to the goal of lasting happiness, freedom from suffering, and spiritual fulfillment. Philosophy does not pay the bills and theories do not comfort the children. After a day of work and family responsibilities, no one has time or energy to sit down and absorb esoteric concepts, so in each chapter the meaning of the Sutra is explained and also applied to specific challenges and stressors we might encounter in normal life. Every chapter ends with Daily Practices, Questions

---

7   Sri Swami Yukteswar Giri, *The Holy Science* (Dakshineswar, India: Yogoda Satsanga Society of India, 1990), 112.

for Further Reflection, and Affirmations that encapsulate the theme to use as inspiring reminders. Instructions on how to accomplish these are included, and it would be helpful to have a journal or notebook handy as you work through this material.

The book's three parts follow the order of the Eight Limbs. Part one covers the first limb called the Yamas, which instruct how to align more completely with our soul nature. Part two outlines the second limb called the Niyamas, which give further practices to integrate our material and spiritual lives. All of these practices have both an internal and an external expression, initiating in our thoughts and inner experience of the world, and then radiating through our words and actions into our outer world. Part three covers limbs three through eight, the deeper ways to address health, energy management, concentration, and finally Self-realization or enlightenment.

The timeless wisdom of these teachings binds together all aspects of who we are as human and spiritual beings, suturing us so that we become integrated and whole. *True Yoga* teaches us how to manage the pressures of working, parenting, and relating, how to live healthy and purposeful lives, and how to ultimately reconnect our souls with Source.

This ancient system of living was not created to give us flat abdominals and the ability to stand on our heads. When we live and breathe our yoga, not just as pretty postures in class but also as real-time practices in every moment with family, friends, and colleagues, we will be happy. *True Yoga* enables us to transform challenge into inspiration, cultivate clarity and compassion, over-come the ego, and develop Self-awareness.

Now it is time to make an important choice. That choice is simply to *be happy*. If we make this one, then no one can stand in the way of our happiness. And if we do not, then no one and no thing can make us happy. The choice and the work are ours alone. I invite you to *choose* happiness *now*. Let us start the journey.

The Eight Limbs of Yoga

Through the practice of the Eight Limbs of Yoga, the
distortions of individual perception are destroyed and the
light of true wisdom brings clarity of consciousness.
Sutra ii.28

Limb One: Yamas: Sutras ii.35–ii.39

Yamas are moral qualities that are necessary for connection to our Soul nature. These behavioral foundations make life more comfortable and spiritually fulfilling as we cultivate relationship with our Self, the world, and the Divine.

Limb Two: Niyamas: Sutras ii.40–ii.45

Niyamas are observances that help us evolve toward harmonious existence within ourselves and with the world, integrating our inner and outer experience. Both the Yamas and the Niyamas state a benefit that we can expect as a result of cultivating that quality or observance.

Limb Three: Asana: Sutras ii.46–ii.48

Asana is the practice of right posture to create physical comfort and ease, eliminate restlessness, and prepare the body to be undistracted in meditation.

Limb Four: Pranayama: Sutras ii.49–ii.53

Pranayama is the regulation and enhancement of the subtle Life Force currents (prana) through which we move into subtler realms of awareness.

Limb Five: Pratyahara: Sutras ii.54–ii.55

Pratyahara is the practice of interiorization of the senses, which develops tranquility and forms a receptive basis for meditation practice.

Limb Six: Dharana: Sutra iii.1

Dharana is concentration or focus. It is training the mind to the single-pointed attention needed for meditation.

Limb Seven: Dhyana: Sutra iii.2

Dhyana is the state of stillness or meditation in which consciousness flows continuously inward rather than outward.

Limb Eight: Samadhi: Sutra iii.3

Samadhi is the bliss of reuniting individual consciousness with the universal One Consciousness.

PART ONE

....

Limb One

....

Inner Work:
Connecting to
Your True
Nature

The complete yoga path is called Raja (Royal) Yoga, encompassing physical and spiritual practices of devotion (Bhakti), service (Karma), and wisdom (Jnana). All of these blend together to support us on our journey to Self-realization. To create a foundation for all of these practices, we begin with the first of the Eight Limbs, the Yamas. Chapters one through five explore five Sutras that describe the qualities necessary for our true spiritual nature to shine forth. These attributes make life more comfortable and spiritually fulfilling as we explore relationship with self, the world, and the Divine.

Yamas translates literally as "abstinences," things we should not do, however the interpretations I offer come closer to the translations given by Nischala Joy Devi in *The Secret Power of Yoga*, in that they focus on the positive quality that should be cultivated rather than what should be avoided. The first Yama on Ahimsa provides an example. The word Ahimsa literally means "non-harming," or "non-violence." But to live a life that is complete and harmonious, we cannot stop with simply *not*

doing harm. We must go the extra mile and develop peacefulness to truly embody Ahimsa in attitude and action. The second quality is truthfulness (Satya), unquestionable integrity in
all circumstances. Third is developing generosity, which again
surpasses Astheya's literal meaning of "non-stealing," because
when we recognize the interconnectedness of all beings, we
perceive the inseparability of giving and receiving. Fourth is
self-control (Brahmacharya), the ability to be moderate and
balanced. And fifth is Aparigraha, translated as "non-greed" or
"non-covetousness." This is expressed as appreciation for what
we have and the awareness of abundance as we acknowledge
the infinitude of creation within and around us. By cultivating
these attitudes, we no longer experience a consciousness of lack.

As these qualities take hold in our thoughts, words, and
activities, we establish a foundation for life that is unshakeable.
When trials come, we have only to look to these five principles of
right living to find the direction in which to go. Choices become
simplified as we weigh them against the Yamas, determining
whether a decision or action brings us closer to this inner alignment or further away. A virtual life compass exists in the first
limb of the Eight Limbs of Yoga.

Each Yama graciously offers both the instruction on development of the quality and the benefit we can expect to receive
when we do. Furthermore, the Yamas set the stage for the deeper
practices of focused attention and meditation that come in part
three. When we have a peaceful mind, a truthful heart, and a

balanced body, we can more easily approach the stillness that expands our consciousness beyond daily reality. These first five directives safeguard our essential happiness.

Chapter One

....

Peacefulness (Ahimsa): Happiness Begins Within

By becoming peaceful, we experience
inner harmony and all outer discord ceases.
Sutra ii.35

Monumental imbalance and strife exist in the world today. There is always something to disturb our peace or make us unhappy. Strangers rage at each other on the road and threats to our safety seem to escalate daily. Conferences on peace take place but individuals still feel alienated and intimidated walking down city streets. The answers to these problems do not exist outside, but rather *within* our own hearts and minds and this is where we begin with the first and most fundamental of the Yamas, the instruction of non-violence (Ahimsa).

World peace will only occur when the world is filled with peaceful individuals; therefore, cultivating Ahimsa or peaceful-ness is our essential starting point. This Sutra indicates that we need to proactively cultivate peace and reverence for all beings, rather than passively remain neutral or non-engaged. Assuming that everything in the Universe is interdependent, each thought and action of every individual affects the overall state of peace and unity in the world. As we make a daily effort to establish harmony within our own hearts and minds, and within our families and communities, we experience the interconnected-ness of all creation and greater love as a result.

This is a practice of profound internal change, and the choice of peace is fundamental to all that lies ahead. If today we choose to live in peace, embracing respect and love for our neighbors, we initiate change not only for ourselves but also for our communities and nations. To evolve in this direc-tion, patient daily willingness to look at our own motivations, agendas, and thoughts is essential.

Moving beyond the traditional translation of "non-harming," we see that Ahimsa means to eradicate anything that undermines peace and to actively start helping. Staying detached is not enough. In order to create harmony where it is not, we must consciously look for ways to practice compassion, respect, and thoughtful-ness each day, first in our thoughts and then in our actions.

To begin, we learn to relax in our own minds and bodies. Rather than curse the people or things that are frustrating us, if we intend to practice peace, we develop the ability to release stress and hold onto behaviors and thoughts that bring us back to serenity again and again. Thought is our greatest ally and creates according to its own nature in both inner and outer results. Therefore, every time we choose thoughts of gratitude, positivity, and peace, we create a ripple of peacefulness on the planet that affects innumerable others. As we manage our stress, frustration, and anger, we offer an example to those around us to do the same.

Thought Watching

To practice the Yamas and Niyamas effectively, we must train ourselves to watch our thoughts. Mindfulness is the ability to be aware of what we are thinking, feeling, and sensing without being pulled around recklessly by it. Watching thought is key to practicing Ahimsa, because all day, every day, if we are not careful and aware, negative thoughts will slip in and chip away at our peace.

Criticism, anger, jealousy, fear, doubt, thoughts of lack, suspicion, and anxiety all negate peace and create inharmony within us. These thoughts act like roadblocks between us and the life of happiness we wish to have. Training the mind to eliminate negativity and concentrate fully on joy and gratitude is essential. At the end of every chapter, affirmations are included to help with the practice of establishing new patterns of thought that will reinforce the qualities we are cultivating. All change begins in the realm of thought.

It is here we enter the labyrinth of intertwining limbs that in their entirety take us to the center of our true nature. Choosing thoughts of peace is the beginning, and the experience of peace beyond thought is also the beautiful outcome of one of the later limbs, that is meditation (Dhyana). The closer we move toward center, the more effective change agents for peace we become in the world.

The Anger Trap

For now, let us start by assessing our outer lives. How often do we react to challenging people or situations in anger? The emotion of anger is meant to spark needed action when controlled, just like a fire is meant to transform wood into productive heat. But unchecked anger, like a fire, will burn out of control in a way that is detrimental to our health—physically, mentally, and spiritually. It is the root of many illnesses as well as premature aging. Uncontrolled anger prevents understanding and our ability to reason clearly.

Consider the expression about giving someone "a piece of our mind." What is actually happening when we tell someone off is that we give away a piece of our inner peace. Let us say that an aggressive driver cuts us off in traffic on the way to work. Whether we roll down the window and yell, or refrain but curse him silently, we have literally given him the *peace* of our mind. Our thought has become poisoned by anger. We are not peaceful. We are not happy. And we are not practicing Ahimsa.

To practice Ahimsa, we stay serene even when conflict arises. We seek a solution based on calm understanding. With the driver who cut us off, we could choose a thought of compassion such as, "He must be really stressed to be driving that way. I hope his day gets better." In doing this, we feel less tension and he receives our peaceful energy waves. Moving away from the problem and toward the solution is key.

Love and calmness are stronger than anger and we must learn to be self-possessed and even-minded under all circumstances in order to move in the direction of happiness. Finding the foundation of peace within the center of our being tethers us to a power far greater than our own. Peacefulness enables us to make wise decisions rather than reactive or ignorant ones. It enables us to stand in the face of conflict or insult unaffected and undisturbed. Ahimsa means giving peace and continual understanding to those who are angry with us until we foster a bridge of harmony.

By the world standard, it is not rational or logical to feel peaceful when confronted, wronged, dismissed, denied, or attacked. Yet it is our challenge to live these spiritual qualities within the challenges of modern life, rather than run to seclusion and avoidance. The Yoga Sutras indicate that by overcoming our ego's desire to justify emotions and engage in conflict, we will move into greater ease and deeper connectivity. By watching emotional reactions arise and choosing *not* to act from them, we are practicing Ahimsa and we experience peace within.

Every frustrating experience of daily life can be approached with either peacefulness or agitation. Part of the practice of Ahimsa is to look within at the ways we choose to remain in conflict and our motivations for doing so. Cultivating peace actively eliminates states of worry and anger.

Both in our thoughts and outwardly in our lives, we will find many opportunities to practice refining more peaceful approaches. Maybe we are holding onto a disagreement with someone, replaying it over and over in our head. Are we harboring resentment or a justification of our position, unwilling to communicate and find compromise? If we cannot harmonize our own minds, emotions, and bodies, we have put ourselves at odds with peace. And even if we are not outright warmongers or conflict instigators, we are contributing to the overall disturbance of anger and fear on the planet.

Let Go of the Need to Be Right

Ahimsa becomes a bit more difficult in family or work situations where feelings and agendas are often intense. What if your partner's work stress is spilling out as short-temperedness with you and the kids? Or a colleague stole a deal you had been fostering for months? It is easy to get angry when we feel mistreated or wronged. We react by attacking back, or putting up an emotional wall. The Sutra on practicing peacefulness is meant for exactly these moments and it requires that we choose the higher, more forgiving and compassionate road even when we might be right or justified in striking back.

Evident by daily news reports, there is plenty of ignorance and hatred in the world that conspires against our effort in this direction. But the choice is ours, moment by moment, in our every thought, word, intention, and action. Clearly, if war were the way to peace we would have achieved it by now.

Mahatma Gandhi, famous Indian political leader and yogi, said that there is no *way to* peace but rather that peace *is the way*. He demonstrated this through his non-violent protests of British rule in India. Through peaceful resistance he withstood violence and successfully effected change for his country, eventually winning even the respect of his enemies.

"Not to hurt any living thing is no doubt part of Ahimsa," wrote Gandhi. "But it is its least expression. The principle of Ahimsa is hurt by every evil thought, by undue haste, by lying, by hatred, by wishing ill to anybody." [8]

The discipline it takes to maintain a mental state of non-violence (Ahimsa) requires tenacity and humility. It is as rigorous as any physical training discipline. The hurt ego is quick to counter. The tired mind is quick to snap. We must slow down and become mindful of our tendencies toward reactivity and judgment. Only then can we create the mental clarity from which to choose wisely, what to say and do that will contribute to peace rather than further conflict. It takes commitment and willingness to stand our ground peacefully, as Gandhi did in the very midst of conflict.

Respect and Care for Self and Others

No peace lies in the future that is not available now, hidden within us in this present moment. It simply depends on our choice. Self-respect and self-care are essential. We are not practicing Ahimsa if we become imbalanced through overwork or

---

8   Eknath Easwaran, *Gandhi the Man* (Berkeley: Nilgiri Press, 1997), 154.

lack of exercise. Practicing Ahimsa is both an inner and outer journey and we cannot offer what we have not embodied. If we feel stressed, unworthy, or afraid then we will create these same feelings in our relationships. When we catch ourselves moving into negative inner spaces, we can remind ourselves of the need for self-honoring in order to contribute to peace on the planet. We can choose thoughts of self-compassion, understanding, and forgiveness, rather than negative thoughts of self-condemnation, criticism, or fear. These thoughts ease our inner experience and we quickly see how transformative this approach can be with others. Ahimsa takes root at our foundation and spreads to all those we encounter.

As we strive to meet all situations and people with loving openness and a dynamic peacefulness, we begin experiencing less stress in our own lives. We let things roll more easily and feel less perturbed when things do not go our way. The more we recognize common needs within all people, the more empathy we feel. We address what lies beneath anger and reactivity, which is usually a deep need for love, understanding, and empathy.

The epic Indian text, the *Mahabharata*, as well as every major religious text since, has encouraged the essentialness of forgiveness under any injury, recognizing it as a noble virtue. Forgiveness releases us from the feeling of anger and the impulse toward retribution, enabling the continuation of harmonious connection between widely differing people, personally and internationally. Whenever we are confronted with opposition, we must conquer with love. Eventually as we eradicate all thoughts that are not peaceful from our minds, we are assured that discord will cease around us. Miracles occur through the creative application of love and forgiveness.

Foundational Happiness

We can all express more love in our thoughts, words, and actions daily. Ahimsa is an active practice that lays the groundwork for all the limbs that follow. By creating an internal environment of peace, watching our thoughts and choosing to hold onto only ones that foster it, and by offering reverence, kindness, and love to all beings, we move toward unity consciousness, the goal of Raja Yoga. If we wish to truly know ourselves and to be fundamentally happy, we must nurture this foundation of spiritual life.

When we are at peace, we are attuned with our soul. As we awaken soul connection, we realize that we are all part of one Divine Essence experiencing life through various human bodies and stories. If we can really feel this oneness, then anything another does is within us as well and we have compassion for him. And anything we do to another, we realize we are doing to ourselves. Every time we take a step in the direction of peace, we effect a positive change in our circle of family and friends. And this extends through them into the greater world.

Never underestimate the power of one peaceful gesture or one peaceful thought. Small steps yield big results over time. If we want to experience peace, we must offer it actively to others. Develop mindfulness and program thought for success and happiness by actively choosing peace at every turn, internally and externally, no matter what happens. Utilize the affirmations at the end of this and every chapter to reinforce the qualities you are developing.

As we embrace forgiveness and choose peacefulness with all beings, we are rewarded with unshakeable inner tranquility and freedom. Our lives move into alignment and our inner light beams brightly. Harmony reigns in our body, mind, and spirit as imperturbable happiness. Eventually all conflict and hostility around us disappear naturally and the world is one step closer to peace.

Daily Practices

Integrate an active practice of peacefulness into your daily life. Remember that it first begins within your own thoughts and then extends to your outer actions. In thought, word, and action, actively choose peacefulness today and notice how even small efforts yield big results over time.

- Watch your inner dialogue. Mindfulness is built one thought at a time. Replace negative, critical, or harmful thoughts with self-honoring, affirming, and loving ones. Write down positive ideas and keep them in a bowl. Reach for one to bring you back to peace when you are feeling angry or upset.

- At breakfast, lunch, and dinner, send a peaceful thought to someone.

- Practice three of the following ways to actively employ Ahimsa today.

  - React kindly even if someone is rude to you.

  - Take time to make eye contact and smile at a stranger.

  - Express gratitude to someone.

  - Make amends to someone you have treated unkindly.

  - Be patient with someone moving slower than you.

  - Send someone who has hurt you a thought of forgivenes.

  - Lend a listening ear to someone who is upset.

  - Yield the right of way to an aggressive driver.

  - Forgive yourself for something.

QUESTIONS FOR FURTHER REFLECTION

Take a moment with your journal now to answer the following questions. Or find a quiet pause sometime today to remember the quality of peacefulness and contemplate these thoughts further.

- How could you practice being more peaceful or respectful with your physical body?

- If you could forgive yourself or someone who has hurt you, would you feel more peace within? Even if you do not know how to forgive in this moment, can you be willing to forgive and see what happens?

- Consider for a moment that whomever you are in conflict with is a reflection of your inner self. How do you hold within you the traits that bother you about them?

- How can practicing understanding and compassion lessen your stress level?

- How does your lack of inner peace contribute to lack of peace in your home or work environment?

Affirmations to Post and Remember

Affirmations solidify beliefs in our subconscious mind, creating a foundation from which we can then manifest positive change in our outer lives. Repeat these often with strong intensity and full faith.

- In my thoughts, words, and actions I practice peace today.

- As I become harmonious inside, perfect peace becomes my experience outside.

- I breathe in peace. I breathe out stress.

- I am peace. Peace is in me.

- I choose to see the Divine within all beings and so I feel harmony with all.

Chapter Two

....

Truthfulness (Satya):
Integrity Creates
Personal Power

When we are established in truthfulness,
our thoughts and words manifest effortlessly.
Sutra ii.36

The second fundamental building block for lasting happiness is integrity. If we are not living from the place of authenticity deep in our heart of hearts, then quite simply we are not living *our* true life. We are living a lie and we will never secure fulfillment materially or spiritually. Truth is powerful and living in truth (Satya) makes us powerful. This Sutra shows how genuine happiness and the ability to manifest our dreams depends on a total commitment to integrity.

Yet, we have all seen untruth used for personal gain and integrity forsaken in the quest for worldly power. From the time we are born, we begin absorbing information, opinions, and beliefs from sources outside ourselves. Influenced by the media, family, friends, and teachers, it is easy to lose track of who we are in an attempt to fit in and stay safe. Through adolescence we may rebel against some of it, but humans need acceptance, so by adulthood we piece together a sense of self built in part on our inner voice and in part on what will be acceptable to those around us. Soon, we find ourselves identified with what is expected rather than what we truly feel and believe.

Living an authentic life can be challenging. What if telling the truth at work compromises our position or authority? What happens when our truth conflicts with a family member's beliefs? How do we even know what truth is if we have just been following the status quo?

Fortunately, by nature, most humans desire to know truth. Eventually the spirit of inquiry that is inherent in us blazes through. Truth is so important that only when we discover it for ourselves and live in full integrity do we feel fulfilled of our unique and joyful purpose. Truth is our compass, our guide to right choices and actions in life and an essential component in our journey to happiness.

Finding Truth in the Body
We begin our connection to truth through the physical body, because it is a great measurer of truth. When we listen within,

we can identify our true feelings based on body sensations. For example, anger might manifest like a tight fist in the belly. Sadness might feel like pressure on the chest, and resentment might feel like heaviness on the shoulders. Once we have an understanding of how our body communicates emotions, needs, and directions, then we have an ongoing gauge of truth.

Take a moment right now to close your eyes and breathe a couple of deep, slow breaths. Imagine a searchlight moving through the inside of your body. When it comes to someplace that hurts or feels tense, hold your attention on that area for a moment and notice any words or images that come to mind. Do these words or images relate to your life in the past, present, or future? Are any emotions attached to these sensations or images?

Our biography lives in our biology. The physical body registers emotional experiences. For instance, if some threat has been a part of our experience, fear will be present in body memory. As a survival mechanism, fear is meant to alert us and get us ready to respond when there is danger. But traumatic fear can leave the body in a state of heightened alertness or protection, which is felt as chronic tension.

As we excavate the truth that lies within sensations, we can decide how relevant the emotional content is today. It may be worth listening to and taking action around, or it may be limiting us and need release. If there is no real-time danger, we can replace stored fear with the truth of the moment. By trusting our bodies, we can let the inner guard down and experience more ease.

Knowledge is power and as we slow down and listen more acutely to the body's way of delivering messages, we attune to a deeper wisdom, an intuitive wisdom that measures how truthfully we are acting and reacting. If we are not living truthfully, we feel isolated and fearful, unable to connect authentically with others. When we move toward truth, listening to our body's raw communication signals, we gain the power to sense what is the right choice or action at any moment of our life. If we notice resistance in the body, we can inquire what the deeper level of truth is in that situation. Maybe we are with someone who is not healthy for us to be with. Conversely, if we are taking a worthwhile risk, we will know it in the very fibers of our physical being.

We can trust our bodies as indicators of whether or not something or someone is genuine. The body is a brilliant guide to both our emotional needs and mental clarity. To know and live the truth, reconnecting with the wisdom of the body is essential.

Bearing Witness to Truth with Compassion

Developing the practice of integrity internally takes courage, because we may not always like what we discover within. If we have been uncomfortable with stillness and self-reflection in the past, it is probably because there is some truth we have not been ready to face. Preferring the convenience of denial or white lies, many people avoid the truth.

We all know the complicated paradox of multilayered truths such as, "I am happy for you *and* I am crushed that you are leaving." Or, "I desperately want this *and* I am paralyzed with the fear of it actually happening." Being honest with ourselves means we can no longer justify our mental laziness or make excuses for our weaknesses.

Truthfulness (Satya) often requires that we make difficult admissions or changes within our lives. It takes courage because in making personal change we expose ourselves to potential rejection if others do not agree or like what we are sharing. Our truth may alienate some of the people we have depended on for our sense of security.

Conversely, we may feel threatened if someone else shares her truthfulness with us and we do not like what we hear. In either direction, compassionately bearing witness to truth is required. Practicing the combination of Satya and Ahimsa, we maintain an open heart rather than indulge the natural tendency to shut down or fire back. We create safe space for each other by listening without judgment, and honoring conflicting feelings. Through Satya we seek understanding regardless of personal feelings, and in mutual vulnerability we build authentic relationship.

Is being honest worth all of the effort and risk? Ask anyone who has lived inauthentically, suppressing their truth or selling out who they are for the sake of a relationship. What is initially undertaken to keep the peace eventually becomes so filled with resentment that any loving motive is obscured.

Although fear of owning and expressing one's truth is common, when we stand courageously forward, we free ourselves. And we enable others to do the same. Satya requires that we be willing to learn through hurt and failure sometimes, to forgive others and ourselves, and to act courageously even when we are fearful. As difficult as these are, ultimately truth is worth it all. It is essential to our inner well-being and to our ability to cultivate real relationships. It is also what gives us the needed direction, vision, and energy to make our lives how we want them to be. When we are firmly established in truthfulness, this sutra says we gain the power of effortless manifestation. Strength and blessings come from the willingness to stand strong in truthfulness.

Finding Truth in Intuition

The next place we must get a hold of truth is in the mind. Often trickier than noticing it in the body, we begin by recognizing that everything we think is *not* true. The mind gathers innumerable impressions daily based on the sensory experiences of life, and merges these with impressions left from the past. These form the basis of inference through which we assume we know what is or will be, based on past conditioning. Relying on sensory perception, inference, and intellectual acuity, we make assessments of what we believe to be true. However, this level of knowing does not carry the same weight as the experience of being one with the truth we are seeking, which comes through the later internal limbs such as meditation (Dhyana).

The Yoga Sutras encourage seekers of truth to go beyond the limitations of intellect to the realization of truth through intuition, perceptible in deep stillness where we find the bridge from individual consciousness to Universal Consciousness through the intuitive faculty. Whereas thought only gives us an indirect perception of truth, intuition gives us the experience of truth from within. This is why, when we intuitively know something, even if the external world cannot prove it, we are sure of its truth.

The Divine essence of truth that the Yoga Sutras describe as being both within and beyond manifestation can only be known through the extrasensory awareness of intuition.

To open the possibility of experiencing truth at this deeper level, we must stop striving for control by defending our beliefs and viewpoints. This requires that we surrender our personal agenda and posturing for success. We practice Satya by letting go of our ego's need to be right, and allow perception to be guided by the Divine within. In direct contrast to the quest for power through manipulation, this approach aligns us with the Infinite Source of true power.

In this way, we achieve an inner congruency in which the soul and the personality work together rather than split with contradictory thoughts and restless feelings. At this quiet place of awareness, when all the other voices around us get still and the mind relaxes, we sit within the deep well of intuitive wisdom, connected to soul consciousness.

To practice Satya, we must attune to this stillness on a regular basis, to feel and know the difference between what is outside and what is inside, and integrate what the head and the heart have to say. Through this integration, we experience more freedom, creativity, productivity, and eventually mastery.

Not All Truth Needs Speaking

This Sutra warns that Satya is so powerful that when we dedicate ourselves to integrity, our thoughts, words, and actions gain the power to manifest. Truth is a dynamic state of mind in which infinite power is released. Of course, with this power comes responsibility. Recognizing that truth is full of consequences, both positive and negative, we acknowledge this power is not to be taken lightly.

The biggest misconception about Satya is that it advocates truth at all costs, and this is not the case. Swami Vivekananda, one of the first Hindu teachers to share yoga philosophy with the West, taught that the practice of intentional peacefulness (Ahimsa) supersedes Satya and therefore moderates the belief that we should share everything all the time without restraint.

Given that this Sutra comes after the one on Ahimsa, it assumes that if we are practicing reverence for all beings, then we understand that telling the truth must be delivered with kindness and sensitivity. We are not meant to be merciless or to serve our self-interest. The essential gauge for whether our truth-telling is necessary lies in our intention.

A bit of self-reflection will reveal the reason *why* we want to share a piece of truth or why we may wish to withhold it. Is it to make us feel superior or vindicated in some way? Truth should only be shared if it is based on a loving intent to foster deeper understanding and harmony. When shared in this way, truth, no matter how difficult, can be healing, balancing, and opening, blessing all the lives it touches. If not, then we need to practice more truthfulness with ourselves about our motivations for sharing. If we discover a hidden agenda that is self-serving in some way, then we should be honest about that. Wisdom and humility are the best guides to right speech.

Ultimately there is one simple criterion for assessing truth that will never steer us wrong. It requires willingness to set aside fear, hurt, desire, and pride in order to know it. The criterion is love. Whatever is anchored in love is truth and we can always trust truth when it is based in love. When we live truthfully from love, we become fearless, free, and able to lead the life that is uniquely ours to live. The practice of Satya delivers us true inner power.

Daily Practice

Integrate an active practice of truthfulness into your daily life. Search inwardly in body, mind, and intuition for the truth and have courage to live into it. Your personal power will increase as a result.

- Listen inwardly to the body and intuition for what you feel is true. Sometimes you will know something before you see proof on the outside. Keep track of confirmations when they come so you can build trust in your inner guidance system.

- Watch your words for a day. Are they kind? Necessary? Peace-inducing? Speak only if they meet all these criteria. Not all truth needs saying.

- Spend a few moments in silence, reflecting on your deepest level of truth about a current issue. Step courageously into speaking and acting from your most authentic place.

- Increase the habit of telling the truth. Notice every time you are about to tell a little less than the whole truth (unless silence is chosen in the spirit of kindness).

Questions for Further Reflection

Take a moment with your journal now to answer the following questions. Or find a quiet pause sometime today to remember the quality of truthfulness and contemplate these thoughts further.

- Where in your body can you sense or feel truth or untruth? Have you ever *known* something was true even before you could prove it?

- Have you ever learned that something you believed was untrue? What is the difference between your opinion and universal truth?

- Reflect upon a lie you have told and how it felt in your body. Why did you tell it? Discuss it with someone you trust and commit to being more truthful from now on.

- How does telling the truth make you free? What would change for you if you lived in total authenticity?

AFFIRMATIONS TO POST AND REMEMBER

Affirmations solidify beliefs in our subconscious minds, creating a foundation from which we can then manifest positive change in our outer lives. Repeat these often with strong intensity and full faith.

- As I live and express my truth, I empower others to live and express theirs.

- I speak my truth with a compassionate heart.

- I am true to my innermost self.

- I share my truth with kindness.

- I live in truth and accept the truth of what is.

Chapter Three

....

Generosity (Astheya): Giving Initiates the Law of Prosperity

When firmly anchored in generosity,
all prosperity comes.
Sutra ii.37

The ability to have our needs met and to manifest rightful prosperity contributes greatly to our worldly happiness. It also indicates our alignment with spiritual law. The key to unlocking the spiritual law of prosperity lies in the Sutra on Astheya. The practice of non-stealing, or to go a step further, the cultivation of generosity, is instructed to assure all material and spiritual success and therefore happiness. Through the awareness of our interconnectedness, we link generous action with truthful intention, and give from what is authentic in our hearts as well as from what is within our physical means. In a balanced exchange of giving and receiving, we experience the intertwining nature of these and the joy that is equivalent in either role.

From the standpoint of non-stealing, Astheya practice calls us to honestly look at the subtle ways in which we take that which is not ours. It could be an idea a colleague had that we spin as our own. Or maybe we copied content from a website that was someone else's creation. It could be taking supplies from the office or taking over conversation when someone else is sharing. Maybe we steal someone else's time by leaving dishes in the sink because we do not feel like washing them.

To practice Astheya authentically, we need to monitor all the little self-serving motives that cross our minds and dictate our choices. Even subtle narcissism has no place in our life if we are practicing Astheya.

Additionally, this Sutra indicates that true fulfillment and prosperity are impossible if we take more than we give on a regular basis. Consider the exchange of giving and receiving in your primary relationships. Do you give more than you take of other people's time, affection, resources, or attention? Do you steal by manipulating them for your desired outcomes? By reflecting on ways in which we take from others on a daily basis, we can make adjustments, and practice offering more than we expect in return. By expecting little from others and much from ourselves, we enter the practice of Astheya.

Selfless Service (Seva)

The yogic practice of selfless service (Seva) exemplifies honest generosity. It encourages us to overcome our egos and personal desires to serve someone else. Everyone can do Seva in some way. We can share our skills, energy, time, patience, and love. If we are capable of monetary offerings, they too should be shared from the standpoint of selfless giving, not so that we may be seen as great and important.

When offered from the heart, Seva brings us joy. It can take innumerable forms limited only by our creativity. Maybe we possess a skill that a friend needs to accomplish a project, so we volunteer some time to help. Or we offer to watch the children of a single parent who is short on time so she can make a yoga or meditation class. We could cook and deliver a meal to someone who is ill or donate a belonging we own that would benefit someone else more than it does us at this time. Recipients of our gestures, whether small or large, will feel love through our thoughtfulness and non-attachment. And we benefit by feeling the happiness of giving.

Tracking Motivation Authentically

To develop a joyful heart through Astheya, we must authentically assess our motivation. We can reflect on questions like these: Am I giving *in order to* receive at a later date, or to obligate the recipient in some way? Am I giving because I feel guilty or unduly responsible for someone else's needs?

If we give because we feel we *should* and not because we are motivated by true caring, then our effort is ego-based and will feel depleting to us and insincere to the recipient. The ego hides in many ways around the domain of giving. We must identify the tricksters of subtle manipulation and selfishness in order to successfully practice the dual elements of honesty and generosity within Astheya.

There are no hard-and-fast rules about how much or how often to give, but one test is always available. Is it motivated by love? The gift of love can be expressed through simple compassion, understanding, thoughtfulness, or empathy. By approaching Astheya in this way, we find many unpretentious yet valuable ways of giving. And regardless of our capacity to give materially, we can always give generously of our love.

Everyone needs to feel loved and it does not deplete us to give love. In fact, the more love we give, the more love we feel within. If we are feeling otherwise, it is time to reflect again on the motivation behind our giving.

Examples of giving from the energy of selfless love are listening with full attention when a friend needs to be heard, or asking about a colleague's well-being with genuine concern. We can offer a hug to a family member in need, or say a silent prayer for a stranger we see struggling. Kindness, attention, and sincere good will benefit others and us.

In the next chapter, we explore the quality of moderation (Brahmacharya), but it is important to note here as well that a fine balance is needed between giving and receiving. We are not meant to over-give to the exclusion of our own self-care and needs. If doing for another jeopardizes our ability to remain in personal balance, then we need to be honest about that with ourselves and with them, and set appropriate boundaries.

If we work a forty-hour week, giving extensively to our employers or clients, it is necessary to practice Astheya with ourselves when the workday is over, generously replenishing our energetic storehouse. If we do too much for our children, we will eventually resent that we have no time for ourselves, not to mention that we do them a disservice by catering to their every whim. The same peacefulness and generosity we show to others we must also give to ourselves. And the same respect and honesty we offer ourselves we must show to all around us.

The Abundant Universe

Giving becomes easier when we realize that we are sustained by an abundant Universe. Infinity is the very nature of the Divine. Aligned with this truth, we feel no lack and therefore no need to take from others. By linking honesty with generosity, making it our practice to give in selfless service at every appropriate opportunity, we experience the benefits of a prosperous heart. The correlation between giving and receiving is a spiritual law. As we give more, in whatever ways we are able, we increase our experience of prosperity in direct proportion. To the degree that we give to others, we attract more of what we need.

If we acknowledge our every breath as a gift from Source, a lightness of being comes into us. We can see ourselves as temporary caretakers of the bodies we inhabit, the children we call our own, and all the material possessions that enhance our lives.

By choosing a mentality of abundance, it becomes easier to accept the changeability of life and the impermanence of all material things. We have been sustained from the time we were born through the generosity of Nature. We can trust the natural abundance that flows to us from Source, providing all that we need. Both inner serenity and outer security are the by-products of Astheya. Without grasping desire, we can remember gratitude and experience an openness that is freeing. We willingly return the favor of generosity through service and love to all.

Blending Astheya with Ahimsa, we perceive the Divine within all beings and the perfect symmetry between giving and receiving. Every moment and every interaction becomes a link between us and Spirit and an opportunity to experience relationship based on unity rather than on self-protection or self-serving. As we open our hearts in generosity, we magnify abundance for ourselves and for all those around us.

Daily Practices

Integrate an active practice of generosity into your daily life. Track your motivations for giving and also your attitudes about provision. Find your personal balance of honest offering in service to the greater good and prosperity will manifest.

- Today, give more than you take, whether it is attention, time, kindness, and so on.

- Practice being generous with your patience. Expect little of others and much of yourself.

- For a week, notice any impulses to give and follow through with them. See how it feels to be free of attachment. Conversely, notice any impulses to withhold and reflect upon how to practice more Astheya.

- Give a gift from your heart, like a hug or a listening ear.

- If you are feeling unable to give, cup your hands like you were going to drink water. This is a gesture of both offering and receiving and is said to reduce the fear of giving. Close your eyes and feel your cup being filled. Then offer it back to Spirit.

- Think of a possession that you have (and value) that someone you know might need more than you do. Consider offering it to them. Notice how this feels different than giving away something you do not want anyway.

- Choose a volunteering opportunity in your community and do not talk about your service. Do it with a quiet presence of selfless service.

Questions for Further Reflection

Take a moment with your journal now to answer the following questions. Or find a quiet pause sometime today to remember the quality of generosity and contemplate these thoughts further.

- Create a list of the ways in which you receive from others. Do you feel grateful and complete and able to return the offering or do you still feel lack? What could you learn from ways other people give to you?

- How can you be a better caretaker of the Earth that generously supports you?

- How could you give more freely of yourself to the world through your relationships, your work, or your talents?

- Reflect on a challenging relationship dynamic you are experiencing. Is the ego harboring a selfish or manipulative motive? If so, could you surrender this and offer love instead?

Affirmations to Post and Remember

Affirmations solidify beliefs in our subconscious minds, creating a foundation from which we can then manifest positive change in our outer lives. Repeat these often with strong intensity and full faith.

- There is always enough for me. I honestly take only what is rightfully mine.

- My generosity creates an open door for me to receive what I need.

- I overcome selfishness by giving first and taking second.

- As I balance giving and receiving in my life, the Universe supports all my material and spiritual needs.

Chapter Four

....

Self-Control
(Brahmacharya):
Moderation
Increases Energy

Dedicated to self-control,
great energy is gained.
Sutra ii.38

Brahmacharya has often been translated as "renunciation" or "celibacy," and for those who have chosen a monastic life, this form of restraint is still their practice. The reason for restricting Life Force Energy (prana) in certain categories of life, such as sexuality, is to have more available for one's growth in another, such as spirituality. But for the everyday yogi or average practitioner, the first step is simply to bring awareness to the habits and desires that deplete us on a daily basis so that we may become more self-controlled in our lives. This ensures that we will have enough inner resources for all that we need to do, both materially and spiritually. Employing balance to find the right levels of work, play, creativity, and service, we moderate the exchange of giving and receiving energy with the world around us.

This Sutra on self-control (Brahmacharya) describes how our storehouse of Life Force Energy will expand exponentially when we cultivate a moderate and balanced approach to life. We utilize prana differently for various activities. In our studies or creative pursuits, we use mental energy. For exercise and household chores, we need physical energy. For relationships and child rearing, we expend emotional energy. To harmonize all of these different ways of engaging with life, we need both vitality and temperance.

More is *not* always better. If we overspend our energy in any one of the above categories, remaining imbalanced for any length of time, we burn out from the accumulated stress that literally turns the internal nature of the body from alkaline to acidic, making it a breeding ground for disease. To maintain health and prevent physical imbalance, it is essential to learn not to deplete ourselves in useless ways, and to let go of unnecessary activities or relationships.

Using Inner Resources Wisely

By looking at energy as a commodity, we can assess where we spend too much or too little. Picture an overview of all the places energy is required: home, work, school, exercise, creative projects, socializing, and spiritual practice. Are some areas monopolizing your energy and some languishing for lack of fuel? We are not necessarily meant to have everything evenly weighted, just properly weighted so we feel peaceful.

Athletes in training know that they must pace themselves over the course of time before a competition. If they were to try to run a full marathon on the first day of training or lift the heaviest weight, they would injure themselves and make it impossible to complete their goal. But if they spread out their workouts and increase their times and challenges appropriately, giving their muscles an opportunity to rest, they increase their capacities and their prana.

The same goes for eating. If we gorge out at one meal, we wind up feeling lousy and sluggish. Our available vital energy decreases as the body uses it to digest and process the excessive food consumed. But if we eat a reasonable portion, then the body converts it to fuel that gives us more energy. Sleep is similar and also needs to be balanced. Too much depletes our energy and makes us feel groggy. The right amount allows us to be renewed and ready for our day.

Self-control applies to the expenditure of effort as well. Greater effort does not necessarily equate to more productivity and it certainly does not equate to more satisfaction. The discernment of how to work smarter not harder applies.

Finally, excessive thinking also needs moderation. Much energy is wasted mulling over the past, worrying about the future, judging what is, trying to be right, and allowing limiting beliefs and fears to affect our choices and actions. Mindful thought-watching and control as explained in chapter one is also an essential part of Brahmacharya as our thoughts can enhance or deplete our energy and creative ability. Fundamentally, the management of our personal energy, both physically and mentally, is one of the best health practices we can employ.

Finding Our Personal Balance Point

By knowing what we want to give our Life Force Energy to, we create priorities. Time with friends and family, time alone, time to get work done, and time to play or exercise all need our attention. If we listen to our bodies, we have an ever-present gauge to see how our personal energy management system is working. If we feel depleted, we will know something is out of balance. If we feel full of energy, we know we are employing the right amount of internal control.

To maintain this, we need to establish daily connection with our inner rhythms and needs. Like nature, which has her cycles of day and night, summer and winter, growing and resting, we also need the rhythms of our lives to be in balanced proportion. When nature's patterns are out of balance, devastation occurs in ways like flooding, drought, or blizzard. When we are off balance, similar chaos occurs in our health, work, or relationships.

We must find our center, our personal balance point. This is the equivalent of engaging our core in a yoga posture. Once we are connected to our center, we can expand outward from there.

In life, this means we prioritize important life goals and say no to extra engagements or tasks that distract us from them. Sometimes it means eliminating relationships that drain us.

To find personal balance, we must remain acutely attuned to each moment, infusing every choice and every action with our full attention. If a parent's needs are not balanced with his children's, he may feel worn thin. If spouses do not maintain both intimacy and individual time, someone will get resentful. When needs are suppressed, we feel our creative Life Force running low. Depression, resentment, or a jockeying for attention shows up or squabbling intensifies.

On the other hand, if we are overindulging our desires, then we are squandering energy potential that we should share with others. By tracking desire with an honest conscience and using self-control, we find the delicate balance point between conflicting familial needs.

The key is to keep the internal scales level. We each have certain things that bring us back to balance. For some people, that is time alone in nature. For others, it might be reading, connecting with a trusted friend, or having a nap. By identifying these, we can regulate our internal equilibrium in the same way the earth does.

The Necessity of Boundaries

Unfortunately, creating balance and practicing moderation are not exactly supported by modern life, in which we are constantly asked and expected to do *more*. Our environments are manipulated with light and technology so we are able to function at all hours of the day and night. The boundaries of home and office, and even of work and vacation, are blurred and we are expected to work anywhere, anytime, because we can. We pay no attention to the seasonal nature of being human, except when the occasional snowstorm shuts down our ability to get to a meeting or school. We live in a culture addicted to adrenaline and the feeling of importance that comes from being busy.

Time management can help us break free and defend our priorities. To start this process, we can ask ourselves: Will I remember this ten years from now? Is finishing something on the to-do list really more important than quality time with my children or partner? If we simplify and prioritize, we create space in both our external lives and in our consciousness. Knowing how we want to use our Life Force Energy on a daily, weekly, and overall life basis, we make choices in energy expenditure that support our goals.

Maybe we have a demanding work schedule Monday through Friday. Having time to play and relax with the kids on the weekend is our highest priority so we keep that in mind when scheduling other commitments. Or maybe we are at home with the kids all week and need time on weekends to get rebalanced through our own creative endeavors. By scheduling the time and space we need to get refreshed, we become more joyfully available to our lives and loved ones. And by giving our full attention to whatever we are doing, we experience an expanded sense of time. We complete tasks more efficiently, with greater results, and feel more in tune with our emotions and more empowered to deal with each situation that arises.

The Happiness of Balanced Living

By human standards, perfect balance is impossible, attestable by anyone who has tried to hold a balance posture in yoga class. Finding equilibrium is hard enough to achieve, much less maintain, for more than five breaths. Too often, we strike a moment of balance, feel great, and then fall out again and spiral into frustration or self-judgment.

Begin by changing that self-negating thought and then move into tune-up mode. Recognize that balance, like any other state of being, is constantly in flux, and create practices to support its gentle maintenance. Scheduling less and maintaining periods of stillness each day give us time and space to equilibrate within. When we turn inward, breathe, and listen we can determine the shifts necessary to bring ourselves back into balance. We can detect illness before it hits and intuit what is needed for the body to heal. We can sense interpersonal dynamics and offer solutions for harmonious interaction. We can respond consciously, rather than react crazily.

Creating balance is never a one-shot deal and sustainability comes through continual adjustment during each new phase of life. The mix is different for a young father with a full-time career and his own creative pursuits or studies than it is for a retired woman committed to charitable or spiritual service.

Whatever stage we are in, managing our prana wisely will give us more energy to use on what is most meaningful, enabling us to infuse every action with intention and our full presence. By practicing self-control and moderation in every aspect of daily living, we gain the energy we need for both our human responsibilities and our spiritual practices. We become more altruistic and less egoistic, able to remain centered and in service at the same time. And we recognize when we shift out of balance and make necessary changes to regain equilibrium.

The practices of self-control and moderation clear away anything that stands between us and the experience of our Infinite Self. We experience heightened creativity, endless vitality, charisma, and a magnetism the yogis call ojas. Literally glowing in our boundless spiritual light, we watch our material life expand exponentially.

Daily Practice

Integrate an active practice of moderation and self-control into your daily life. By consciously monitoring the expenditure of your Life Force Energy, you will be able to make wise choices for personal balance.

- Like your money, your energy account needs a budget. Notice where your personal energy management system needs rebalancing. Set appropriate boundaries.

- Everyone has preferred rhythms of eating, sleeping, working, resting, and reflecting. Make changes to honor your favored daily rhythms.

- Check in periodically during your daily activities and ask yourself if what you are giving your time and attention to will matter in ten years. Prioritize the use of your precious Life Force Energy.

- Make a list of all the projects you have that are incomplete. Decide whether you still wish to complete them. Commit a specific time frame to those that you do. Mentally delete the others. Employ self-control to accomplish your goals.

Questions for Further Reflection

Take a moment with your journal now to answer the following questions. Or find a quiet pause sometime today to remember the quality of moderation and contemplate these thoughts further.

- Draw a circle and divide it into pie-like slices that represent your energy expenditure in all the major categories of life, such as work, education, exercise, family time, hobbies, creative projects, friends, community service, spiritual practice, and rest. The sections that you give the most energy get the bigger slices and those given the least energy get smaller slices. Are there imbalances? What needs to shift so that you can have more prana available for the important slices of life?

- What or who drains your vital energy physically, mentally, or emotionally? How do you overspend your energy?

- How much time do you use thinking about the past? Try letting those thoughts go and putting that energy into creating something better in your life today.

- What signals does your body send when you are nearing depletion or close to your tipping point? Consider what your body needs to feel more balanced right now. More sleep? Less alcohol? Different diet? More fresh air?

- In what way do you need to practice more self-control?

Affirmations to Post and Remember

Affirmations solidify beliefs in our subconscious minds, creating a foundation from which we can then manifest positive change in our outer lives. Repeat these often with strong intensity and full faith.

- Standing on the scale of balance, I listen to my body and make daily adjustments for peace and harmony.

- I live from my priorities.

- I effortlessly balance time with family, work, others, and myself.

- Balance and moderation in all things bring me ease and vitality.

- Self-control enhances my Life Force Energy.

Chapter Five

....

Appreciation (Aparigraha): Gratitude Brings Abundance

Overcoming envy and fear, we cultivate
appreciation and understand
the true purpose of our life.
Sutra ii.39

The Universe is an ever-renewing, infinitely creative field of pos-
sibilities. Abundance exists all around us all the time. Yet we often
keep our vision so trained on the tiniest speck of reality that we
block the flow of this unlimited potential into our minds, hearts,
and lives. We declare lack and focus on what we do not have
instead of affirming plenty and giving gratitude for all that we do
have. Such limiting beliefs and narrow perceptions cause us to
suffer. They also perpetuate the experience of deficiency. When

we remember that the wellspring of all resources is inexhaustible, and we place ourselves into its loving stream, we receive an outpouring of goodness, joy, beauty, opportunity, support, guidance, and creativity.

The consciousness of appreciation (Aparigraha) magnifies our happiness. Regardless of material possessions or success, we cultivate this state of mind by acknowledging the blessings all around us and recognizing opportunities for growth through every circumstance. In this way we eliminate greed and covetousness and move closer to the Source of true fulfillment. We recognize Spirit as our constant storehouse of supply.

The key to having this experience is to understand that both gratitude and abundance are cultivated attitudes. They are not dependent on the actual outer provisions or circumstances we have at any given moment. It is our *belief* in abundance or the lack thereof that creates our experience of it. And our ability to be grateful for what is present is exactly that which brings more goodness to us—just like a fearful belief will often magnetize to us that which we fear.

Practicing an abundance mentality means noticing when and how we feel limited mentally and actively nurturing the opposite thought in those moments. For instance, if we feel time-limited because of overcrowded schedules, we can proactively affirm the limitless nature of time, and practice being more present moment by moment. We can talk back to the voice in the mind shouting about not getting things done, and trust the infinitude of time. If we are repeating thoughts about material lack, we should affirm our creative ability to manifest new ideas and ways of solving the problem, and pause to appreciate the many material blessings that we have in this moment.

Opportunities Abound

By looking for blessings within every situation, every experience, and every encounter, we become empowered to deal with challenge differently. Even when we are frustrated or struggling, we have an opportunity for personal growth that offers us value in the long run. Take for example a relationship filled with conflict and misunderstanding. If we approach it as a place where we can learn how to be more compassionate with the other person and with ourselves as we attempt resolution, we grow wiser and stronger. If we approach the mounds of work on our desk or the emotionally charged meetings with a perspective of curiosity and creativity, rather than just as a threat to our serenity, we find an endless drawing board for self-development. Instead of being afraid or pushing difficulty away, we embrace it as a gift from the abundant Universe.

This requires a true paradigm shift much like the old proposal, "Is the glass half empty or half full?" It requires trust and willpower and the choice of a positive attitude at all times. But this is the magic of this Sutra. By choosing to acknowledge abundance and blessings, even when things are not exactly as we would like them to be, an amazing thing happens. We open ourselves to the gracious flow of Universal energy.

If we hold on or hold back, we impede this flow. Holding back comes from the belief that we do not, or will not, have enough time, resources, validation, support, and so on. This fear leads to mental restriction, a lack of generosity, and unavailability to life. As with the practice of generosity (Astheya), this requires a leap of faith sometimes, when we outwardly have little to spare or share. But practicing Aparigraha establishes a free-flowing exchange with life where we receive and give in balance and ease.

The correlation is notable. The more generosity we practice, the more abundance we experience. The more we realize abundance, the more generous we become. Although outwardly we may feel we have little, by seeing the glass half full, we bypass perceived lack, and the ways in which we do have abundance are revealed. The thrilling truth is that when we start appreciating all that is and looking for abundance, it appears everywhere.

Accumulation and Obligation

Studies on happiness have shown that it is not determined by material wealth and comfort. In fact, the more dependent we become on externals for our happiness, the less we actually experience satisfaction from them. The fear of loss that quickly follows the acquisition of something external affects the mind in negative ways, keeping us in a constant state of dissatisfaction. Seen in the unhappiness of many wealthy people, fear is an insidious enemy that corrupts our peace and prevents us from finding fulfillment in this moment and joy in the very things we have acquired.

Fear limits our ability to practice appreciation and perceive abundance. And in the fear of not being able to get or retain what we feel is enough, we end up taking too much, creating the further destructive habit of wastefulness. We observe this with children whose "eyes are bigger than their bellies." But as adults we all have our ways of grasping in the same fearful way. Think of all the things you own right now that are unused and unneeded. The yoga teachings caution that greed and covetousness arise if we do not put a cap on our desires for and accumulation of physical goods.

Greediness or hoarding is a form of insecurity, the need to fill up from the outside rather than know from the inside that we *are* and that we *have* enough. This Sutra is not instructing us to be complete renunciants or to take a vow of poverty. It is simply cautioning us to monitor both our motivations for acquisition and our attachment to that which we acquire. Just because a new version of a product is available does not mean it is necessary. Over-accumulation often places us into debt, financially and energetically, in obligation to organizations, people, and things. The Sutra on Aparigraha warns that we restrict our mental freedom by receiving or purchasing anything that bears indebtedness as a result.

The ability to differentiate between desires and needs is essential for the aspiring yogi. We can practice limiting desires and appreciating the things we do have as a custodian rather than as an owner so as not to build identification and attachment to material items. Whether we have much or little, practicing the attitude of abundance will release us from the grip of fear and lack.

The Promise of Purpose

By having less physical possessions to preserve and maintain, we liberate time and energy. And by watching our interpersonal motives for giving and receiving, we become more balanced in our relationships. We discover a wellspring of energy that we can devote to what matters most in life, like determining what we are here to express or how we are meant to serve the needs of the world through our unique skills and perspectives.

Like all the Yamas, this Sutra on Aparigraha offers a distinct benefit that comes from reducing desires and accumulation while holding a perspective of appreciation within. As we magnify the love in our hearts through the perspective of abundance, we receive the benevolence of life and the understanding of our greatest sense of purpose, that which will bring us true fulfillment and more happiness than any material possession.

The outer practices of self-control (Brahmacharya), generosity (Astheya), and truthfulness (Satya), combined with the cultivation of appreciation (Aparigraha), create a fertile field within us, ready for the inner practices of yoga that lie ahead in part three. By devotional surrender of material attachements, we prepare the mind to develop deeper concentration (Dharana) and stillness (Dhyana).

The Abundance of True Self

Suffering is inevitable as long as we grasp outwardly for things to fill us up and make us feel better. But when we turn inward and acknowledge Spirit as the origin of all our resources, we find the inexhaustible joy of our true nature. All the love, creativity, and wisdom we need are there, and we fully and finally quench the longings that we have sought through outer pleasures. The entire teachings of the Yoga Sutras point to this realization as the goal of practice.

Through Aparigraha, we know that we are complete as we are right now, perfect in our spiritual essence. There is no need to grasp or cling to anything outwardly in order to be whole. We hold an inner richness that is always there, even when it is temporarily obscured by the clouds of stress or challenge. We see the blessings in every difficulty, every loss, every success, as well as every setback. And we develop a consciousness of abundance that enables us to define with joy the course and intention of our lives.

DAILY PRACTICES

Integrate an active practice of appreciation and gratitude into your daily life. By watching for the opportunities and blessings in all circumstances, we get clearer about what we have come to learn and share in this lifetime.

- Take some silent moments to open your heart today to the abundant blessings in your life. Feel and express gratitude to anyone you encounter. This can be simultaneously simple and profound.

- Practice "positive flooding." Tell someone you care about everything you think is wonderful about him or her. You can also practice appreciating yourself in this way.

- Remember Astheya (generosity) and notice how the more you give, the more abundance you perceive.

- Take stock of your current possessions and release any that hold the energy of greed, fear, or obligation.

Questions for Further Reflection

Take a moment with your journal now to answer the following questions. Or find a quiet pause sometime today to remember appreciation and contemplate these thoughts further.

- Watch your thoughts, opinions, and beliefs. Do they ebb and flow freely or do you hold them tightly?

- Notice whether you hold a mentality of limitation or abundance. How does this affect your happiness and life?

- Create an abundant ABC list. For every letter, think of something you have to be grateful for.

- Before buying anything new, ask yourself, "Is this a desire or a need? Does this have a true purpose or am I just accumulating out of lack mentality or greed?"

- Imagine the most amazing possible purpose for your life. What talent, skill, or resource do you have that can serve the world today?

AFFIRMATIONS TO POST AND REMEMBER

Affirmations solidify beliefs in our subconscious minds, creating a foundation from which we can then manifest positive change in our outer lives. Repeat these often with strong intensity and full faith.

- I am richly blessed by the abundance of this day.

- With gratitude, I accept whatever the Universe offers me today.

- I immerse myself in the flow of Divine abundance now.

- I open to receive freely from the Source of all abundance.

- I align with my highest purpose, trusting its unfolding as I cultivate an attitude of appreciation and gratitude.

Life Integration: Creating a Harmonious Existence

In chapters six through ten, we explore the second of the Eight Limbs of Yoga called the Niyamas. The five Niyamas are observances that lead us toward harmonious existence within ourselves and with the world. They are practices that integrate our material and spiritual lives, accelerate our evolution, and take us ultimately to liberation. It is necessary to cultivate the Niyamas in order to be available for the internal quests of energy control and meditation found in part three.

The Niyamas are a combination of attitude and action. Developing purity (Saucha) and contentment (Santosha) have internal and external expressions manifesting in our thought and actions. The commitment to right behavior (Tapas) begins within and extends into our life choices. Self-study (Swadhaya) applies to what is individual and as well as to what is Universal. And devotional surrender (Iswara Pranidhana) is only accomplished when it is first deeply anchored in one's loving heart.

Like the Yamas, each Niyama summarizes the desired practice to develop, as well as the benefit we can expect to receive when we do it with consistency. These are not quick fixes but standards to move toward over the course of a lifetime. Their application to daily circumstances becomes ever more apparent as we open our awareness to how the Niyamas affect us at every turn in our journey. Like varied spices in a recipe that blend impeccably into a delectable dish, these observances change the flavor of our lives to an ever more soulful palette.

When the combined practice of all ten Yamas and Niyamas is integrated into the fibers of our being, we will be soul-centered and ready to move into a broader understanding of the purpose of yoga and life.

Chapter Six

....

Purity (Saucha): Choosing Less Offers More

By cultivating purity of heart, mastery
over the senses and one-pointed thought are achieved.
Then one becomes fit to behold the Soul.
Sutras ii.40–ii.41

Purity comes through simplicity. Simple living means we choose to have and do less, but as a result we enjoy more. By clearing out things that make our lives and minds too busy, we purify our inner landscape, honoring what is most important. When we create more space to breathe, imagine, and listen to the longings of our hearts and souls, this Sutra on purity (Saucha) assures us that we will find deeper Self-awareness and complete joy.

Theoretically, simplification sounds good to most people but figuring out how and where to begin is challenging. Stress is at an all-time high in the world today. Seventy-seven percent of people polled report feeling symptoms associated with tension and anxiety *regularly*, according to a 2014 study by the American Psychological Association at the American Institute for Stress. [9] These feelings of stress lock the parasympathetic nervous systems into the production of cortisol and heighten our body's fight-or-flight response. When we run on this kind of adrenaline for an extended period of time, we become physically and mentally unable to relax and slow down. Our immune systems become compromised and stress-induced illnesses develop. Eventually we collapse.

Purity and simplicity, however, seem counter to modern reality. We live in a culture of insatiable consumerism, where advertisements push us constantly toward the newest, fastest, biggest, and most prestigious. We increase the complexity of our lives by adding more and more to our plates, acquiring and multitasking at an epic level. Almost every daily choice has become complex. How many social media outlets can we maintain? Which of the thousands of supplements for optimal health should we take? Where on the oversaturated Internet can we find needed information? Even spiritual seekers who intellectualize the need for simplification complicate their search for Self-knowing through an endless stream of trainings, podcasts, retreats, and workshops.

---

9   American Psychological Association, American Institute of Stress. http://www.statisticbrain.com/stress-statistics/. Accessed July 8, 2014.

The Calm within the Storm

This Sutra on Saucha does not instruct us to sell our worldly possessions or to go live on a secluded mountaintop. Nor does it glamorize some nostalgic ease of days gone by. Practicing Saucha means functioning in the complexity of the world while staying connected to and identified with the pure Self within. This is our peace in the eye of life's storm. It supports the clarification of our priorities mentally, physically, and emotionally in order to reclaim our natural state of happiness. It anchors us in our innate joy that is not dependent on outer circumstances.

Deep wisdom and serenity lie in simplicity. Profound experience exists in one fully present breath. We have to slow down to realize that less actually brings more. But simple is not the same as easy and anything worthwhile takes practice.

Many people have lost the ability to orient themselves within. They have become toxically associated with what they *have* and what they *do,* rather than who they *are.* This materialistic focus keeps us forever on the treadmill of acquisition and achievement, for the sake of maintaining the ego's false identity or status. But we are seeking identity and fulfillment in the wrong places.

If we succumb to the incessant urges to buy, consume, and attain, we build a self-imposed jail of material items that then requires more time and energy to maintain. The greater the ego's attachment to possessions the greater its fear of their loss and the more need it feels to protect and defend. Material acquisition becomes habitual, even addictive to some, as they continually seek happiness from the outside rather than within. No amount of possessions will ever bring lasting fulfillment.

In addition, our activities can also become excessive. Saying yes to every social engagement or project, filling every moment, is not efficient and will not produce true enjoyment. By limiting the number of activities we undertake, we create more quality time for those we do participate in. If, on the other hand, we are forever moving on to the next task or distraction, we do not have a chance to digest and assimilate what has transpired. Just as if we ate continually throughout the day, our bodies could not assimilate and eliminate the food efficiently.

Saucha tells us that it is time to give our bodies and minds a rest from the incessant intake. We need to purify the mental and the physical landscapes of our lives. Even during a busy day we can find spaces to pause. We do not need to check our phones every other minute. If we are waiting in a line, we can just relax and let free thought drift through. Rather than overscheduling our children, we can teach them to be satisfied with just one structured activity per season, leaving time for imaginative play.

The Gift of Boredom

People who feed on the rapid-fire pace of modern life are often afraid to be still for fear of falling behind, feeling deprived, or getting bored. Even the word "simple" may hold a boring or blasé connotation to some. Unfortunately, we have collectively forgotten the gift that boredom brings, which is the gift of creativity. As we move from a state of reaction to one of reflection, we are able to see more of who we are and how we can live more intentionally.

Simplification offers psychic space where our minds can meander, imagine, make new connections, and think new thoughts rather than the same, repetitive old ones. With less to do, we can be more inspired and insightful. Boredom invites us to the pure field of inner resourcefulness.

When we have fewer forces pulling at us, it is easier to stay centered. We hear what our hearts and souls have to say and find the conviction to make necessary changes. The dictionary defines simplicity as "easily understood or done, presenting no difficulty." Imagine if today was full of ease and presented no difficulty? Choosing simplicity can help make it so.

In the pure moments of presence, we receive deep pleasure as well. A much-needed hug, eye contact, a listening ear, someone holding a door when our hands are full, all bring us simple joy. When we slow down enough, we realize that doing and having less actually brings deeper fulfillment.

We can begin immediately by eliminating one thing from our to-do list. One thing. There has to be something that is not essential. And we can practice being completely present to whatever activity or person we are with rather than multitasking. When we focus on one thing at a time, we create a more easeful experience and a fuller connection in relationship.

Simplifying Thought Purifies the Mind

More challenging than simplifying on the outside is simplifying on the inside in our own minds. If only we could turn thought *off* without going to sleep or using an escape mechanism like television, Internet surfing, or alcohol. In chapters thirteen and fourteen, the practices of sensory withdrawl (Pratyahara) and concentration (Dharana) help us do just this. Replacing the agitation of overload with peaceful purity and focus helps us let go.

Think of a concern you have been mulling over mentally. Imagine placing this worry or challenge in a container, sealing it, and setting it aside. You can reopen it whenever you choose to, rather than allow it to wildly overtake your mental space without your permission. In this way, we create inner space and find that we can relax, instead of lying in bed at night repeatedly thinking about a distressing conversation or some unfinished business.

When we are relaxed and purified in the tranquility of Saucha practice, an amazing thing happens. We discover what makes us feel alive and creative, imaginative, and purposeful. We discover who we are meant to be in this moment, instead of what the world is shouting at us to be. We find intuitive answers to the questions that have been plaguing us. We find within a deep well of truth (Satya).

By eliminating clutter in both our outer environment and in the inner landscape of thought, we refine our lives. As we relinquish attachment to the stuff that accumulates physically and mentally, we become free. Inertia, lethargy, doubts, mental fatigue, and distraction are replaced by understanding, focus, confidence, positivity, and patience.

The clearer we become mentally, less invested in defending a false identity based on material status or possessions, the easier it is to laugh at the inevitable pitfalls of being human. When we can bring mental and emotional levity and even humor to life, it feels like a breath of fresh air. A lighthearted perspective eases tension and allows for empathetic awareness to bloom. Consciously choosing a positive, enthusiastic attitude is the greatest help to removing the mental and emotional obstructions within that alienate us from our innate wisdom and joy.

Centered in Simplicity

Being centered in our true, purposeful nature feels calm and detached but still present and engaged. Emotional charge is gone but we are fully available to the relationship or process at hand. It is radically different from being disconnected, which happens when we give up through emotional or physical withdrawal.

Maintaining a centered awareness requires that we learn to fully relax with whatever is happening around us. We employ Brahmacharya to manage our Life Force Energy. We practice Aparigraha to expand our experience of joyful abundance through appreciation, and because we feel good, we naturally offer Astheya through greater willingness to serve or give to others. Our personal power remains anchored in Satya and we live in the peaceful acceptance of Ahimsa.

As we release mental obstacles like judgment, fear, arrogance, or self-pity, exchanging them for simple spiritual awareness, we reorient toward the Divine Self that is within. Our well-being and performance levels increase and we reduce stress and anxiety-related illness. From this grace-filled place, we make choices for a balanced life and we rise above any challenge through the purity of love and wisdom.

DAILY PRACTICE

Integrate an active practice of purity and simplicity into your daily life. By eliminating non-essentials, going against the societal trend of more equals better, we create space for what brings ultimate purpose and fulfillment to our lives.

- Eliminate one activity this week. Continue until the level of activity in your life feels simple and manageable.

- Make a list of simple pleasures, things that cost little or nothing. Make a date to enjoy one this week.

- Get rid of possessions that are not used regularly. Start with one room and go from there.

- Find a natural object that appeals to you, like a shell, a stone, or a leaf. Place it on a table all by itself in your home or office. Appreciate how much more you see in it when it is by itself. When you are feeling busy or overwhelmed, stop and stare at this natural beauty. Breathe deeply for a few minutes. Then close your eyes and see it in your mind's eye. Feel your body start to relax.

- Create a space of purity in your home or office and do not let anything invade it. Let it remind you of how clearing space within your mind makes room for the joyful you to come through.

QUESTIONS FOR FURTHER REFLECTION

Take a moment with your journal now to answer the following questions. Or find a quiet pause sometime today to remember the quality of purity and contemplate these thoughts further.

- Consider a situation in your life that feels complex. What is the simplest meaning and the simplest solution you can imagine?

- Notice a desire you have. On the spectrum of want versus need, where does it fall?

- Practice this acronym or make up your own:

  - S: Stop

  - I: Inquire

  - M: Be Mindful

  - P: Be Present

  - L: Listen

  - E: Enjoy

- If you are trying to do three things at once, do you do any of them well? How does simplicity support your creativity?

- What brings you the purest joy? How do you receive more from less?

Affirmations to Post and Remember

Affirmations solidify beliefs in our subconscious minds, creating a foundation from which we can then manifest positive change in our outer lives. Repeat these often with strong intensity and full faith.

- By practicing simplicity, I make room for what matters most.

- The purest things bring the most joy.

- My life becomes happier and less complicated as I practice simplicity.

- When I choose simplicity I expand creatively.

- Simplicity reveals true purpose.

Chapter Seven

....

Contentment (Santosha): Accepting What Is Equals Freedom

Through contentment
ultimate happiness is achieved.
Sutra ii.42

There are certain things we can change in life and certain things we cannot. The Sutra on contentment (Santosha) encourages us to discern the difference and to be in harmony with what *is* through peaceful acceptance. This does not mean passivity or lack of action. Rather, it is disciplined self-control, and the regulation of desire in order to appreciate what we have now, instead of restlessly seeking, or reactively critiquing others or ourselves in some way. Practicing Santosha brings us to peace and joy in this very moment.

But what if things are really going wrong? How can we be content with losing a major contract? Or with four hours of sleep? Or with having to renegotiate child support *again*? With so much in life that needs doing and fixing, practicing contentment may seem like a cop-out. Let us be clear. Choosing to be content no matter what does not mean being unresponsive. It just means that we relinquish all expectations that things will be different than they are, *and* at the same time be willing to work for positive change with non-attachment. It also means we continue training our minds to see the positive blessing in any and all circumstances as discussed in the chapter on Aparigraha.

Like all the Yamas and Niyamas, this Sutra has subtle layers of meaning. Santosha offers a perspective on finding peace within the chaos of modern life. It is human nature to strive, create, and achieve. *How* we move into action and toward change is the challenge.

Resistance Causes Suffering

The simplest way to begin is to stop complaining about the things that annoy us and gently accept the things that fall short of our desires. We all know life does not always go our way. If we find humor in what otherwise might make us crazy, life becomes a little lighter. For example, if we spend our morning commute cursing at the "idiot drivers" on the highway, we arrive at work enraged. But if we spend it noticing the wildflowers blooming on the side of the road, we arrive with patience intact and a more positive frame of mind to start the day.

Maybe we just want to run in the store for a quick morning coffee but cannot find a parking spot. This can be an opportunity to be content without coffee and cut down on caffeine. If we do not get our expected promotion, we can practice acceptance and look for new ways to grow creatively in our current position. If the kids are acting out, we can practice serenity while assessing new solutions. All of the experiences we encounter in life are just material to use in various ways, like raw clay that can be molded into a variety of shapes.

It helps to recognize that anything we are struggling against in non-acceptance causes us to suffer. Most of the time, the question "why," as in why is this or that happening, is not helpful and actually locks us into an internal place of struggle. If we do not want to experience so much anguish, then we can approach all experiences life delivers as opportunities for our growth and understanding.

No Victims

Sometimes life delivers a more severe blow. We are beset by unexpected tragedy, random negativity, or cruel treatment from another. Maybe someone we love gets hurt or dies. Although we may not have control over difficult circumstances happening now, we do have a choice about how we react to them.

To understand the nature of Karma is helpful. From the Sanskrit root *kri*, meaning "to do" or "to make," Karma is the correspondence of every action and its equal and similar reaction, either now or in the future. Yogic philosophy supports the belief that everything we are experiencing now is a result of our own actions in this or some past life. Karma is a natural law, like gravity, that we cannot avoid. We feel its effects daily.

The principle of Karma itself is not positive or negative, but each of our actions has either a positive or negative consequence. Karma does not come to punish us but to teach us that everything that is happening is a current opportunity to evolve spiritually through our chosen reaction. When we stop focusing on situations as bad or good, we free up a tremendous amount of energy that can be used in more intentional ways, such as finding what we can learn from the situation and how we can become stronger rather than holding a victim consciousness.

In this way, we use our energy for a higher purpose and we move in the direction of true contentment (Santosha). It is draining to remain in a state of victim mentality. It disempowers us and prevents us from finding meaning in life. How we respond to difficulty determines whether we continue suffering or rise to victory in this present moment. It also determines whether we set up positive or negative Karma for the future. By remembering to practice Santosha when Karma hits us, we accept what is beyond our control to change and we use our free will and creative abilities to respond productively to what we can change.

Cultivating an attitude of acceptance and willingness to use each experience for our spiritual and personal development does not mean we choose non-action in the face of injustice. But we do eliminate resentment for what we must face and establish a calm ability to walk through any circumstance with a peaceful heart. By trusting the process of life in its entirety, we begin to make wise, self-honoring choices from a centered place of clarity and conviction. Far from easy, keeping our hearts open while being challenged from every side is one of the most exhaustive practices in the Sutras, and one of the most rewarding.

Contentment with the Body

An interesting and necessary place to practice Santosha is in our attitude toward our physical bodies. We were all given certain physical attributes, some of which we may not like. And although we would all like to be perfectly fit, flexible, and balanced, that may be out of reach for some. By giving the body respect and honor, it will open, strengthen, express, and release in ways that would be impossible if we just tried to force it into submission. If we choose compassion and acceptance for our body today, we enable its innate power of healing, reprogramming, and awakening. With acceptance, we come home to ourselves, breath by breath, movement by movement.

To begin, reflect on how you treat your body. Do you demand too much, or do you pay little regard to proper health practices? How do you treat others physically? And how do you allow others to treat you? If we do not like what we discover in this reflection, a deeper commitment to integrating the practices learned in earlier Sutras, like honesty, peacefulness, and moderation, can be helpful in combination with self-acceptance.

A large part of Santosha practice is suspending the constant inner commentary that usually goes on in the mind. Judgment and criticism stoke a larger fire of unrest within that separates us from our true Self and from love. If we want to feel joy, we must mindfully watch our thoughts and redirect them when they err toward negativity. What does it matter if our friend gained twenty pounds, or a neighbor plays strange music, or our latte is not made to perfection?

Judgment is the great wall that divides us, from others and from ourselves. It causes pain and separation and it prevents us from living peacefully. Contentment, on the other hand, creates healing and loving relationships.

As we choose to accept what is and make it okay to be how and who we are, we also allow others to be how and who they are, right now. This is the very essence of mindfulness, being with what is right here, right now, bringing our *full* attention to each moment. Through single-pointed focus we release expectation and fear. Fear closes us off. Love makes us receptive to whatever is. Deep trust allows us to let go of expectation, and we feel content in our bodies as well as in relationship to others. By eliminating fear and preconception of how we think things should be, an enhanced sense of inner tranquility and well-being becomes ours.

According to the Sutras, we should care for our physical form, but find our true identity with the soul that lives within. If we change our perception of self from body to soul, we see beyond the limited physical expression and are therefore less disturbed by its challenges and changes.

Contentment in Failure

Failure is as much a part of life as success. Yet humans fear being seen in our imperfection. Our children might lose confidence in us or our employees may question our authority. Without a doubt, it is important to model strength and expertise, but there is value as well in failing gracefully and using failure productively. Again it is *how* we undertake challenge and change.

To gain true strength, we need to acknowledge our limitations and share how we are working to improve them. When we openly own our failures in conjunction with new efforts to advance, people respect us more because we demonstrate how failure is just a part of the path and not the end of the road. Self-acceptance helps us take a first step toward changing in a positive direction and empowers others to do the same. Contentment is an ever-active practice and should not be confused with complacency or stagnancy.

As we forgive our own weaknesses and failures, we allow others to accept theirs with dignity as well. If we model honesty, explaining our mistakes and the learning we received as a result, then apologies can be made and conflict can be released through mutual forgiveness. The more our friends and families see us employ this loving release, the more they will feel comfortable doing it too. Condemnation does not help us, or anyone, in achieving aspirations. We must establish a new dialogue inside our minds, and with our peers, one that speaks with compassion and acceptance, rather than blame and judgment.

Ever Willing to Change

Santosha practice encourages us to be mindfully content during the journey, not just at the destination. We can still make goals and take steps to accomplish them. But if we achieve one and then immediately expect more or feel guilty for what we have not yet accomplished, we are no longer practicing Santosha.

As we do what is in our power today to move closer to our goals, and then surrender into the practice of contentment, we can rest easy. Rather than fear the fact that we cannot control the future, we can take comfort in the fact that all we must do is accept and deal with what is happening now. Tomorrow will inevitably bring a changing set of circumstances and accepting those circumstances will be our work for *tomorrow.*

Without having big personal agendas and expectations weighted in the past or future, we free up tremendous energy for this moment. We feel lighter. And we get more out of whatever is happening because we participate with it completely instead of splitting our focus and energy into two or more places.

Attachment (Raga) and Aversion (Dvesa)

Consider how, when life is perfectly aligned, we try to hold tightly to the circumstances of that time, place, or person. We do not want anything to change because we finally feel so good. This is the state of attachment (Raga). Yet life is constant change and everything material is temporary, so if we are attached then we suffer when it ends. Similarly, if we resist unpleasant circumstances in life, bemoaning why something is happening that we do not like, we suffer from the state of aversion (Dvesa).

The secret of happiness lies in non-attachment to anything changeable. We can enjoy sensory pleasures but remain free by carrying always a consciousness that extends beyond the material realm. Herein lies the difference between short-lived satisfaction and the contentment and peace that withstands time and space.

By embracing life as a grand play we can see that, like actors on stage, we have choices. If we focus on what is wrong, we remain in constant discontent. If we identify with the Divine within, nothing can come between us and joy.

As we embody Santosha, we become less compelled to react, fix, analyze, change, or manipulate. We assess desires by whether something will take us closer to or further from inner peace and contentment. We ask ourselves questions to determine if something is a transitory or a lasting pleasure. Is it necessary? Is it for my highest good and the highest good of all beings? Will it bring me enduring happiness? If we determine it to be a good choice, then we can move forward while at the same time offering our enjoyment to the Divine.

Having a sense of humor helps us do this. And smiling even when we do not feel happy is a powerful way to bring ourselves back to a lighthearted state of mind. We cultivate Santosha by seeing things in a positive light and seeking a reason to be happy rather than defending why we should be unhappy. In this way, we move toward the state of supreme joy that this Sutra promises is the outcome of Santosha.

Contentment is a dynamic attitude that calms the mind, establishing it firmly within the essence of our true nature rather than the constantly shifting outer environment. By cultivating this mental well-being, we establish a foundation for genuine self-confidence and success in all our personal endeavors. Through our choice to be content no matter what, we claim the power to be happy and free. And we become receptive to the Infinite moving into manifestation through us in ever-changing form.

Daily Practice

Integrate an active practice of contentment into your daily life. Notice all the ways in which opinion or struggle arises and practice letting go of the constant quest for your personal agenda. Open to learning through all that life brings.

- If something is not to your liking, or you are feeling challenged in some way, practice smiling through your eyes. See something beautiful around you and beam a good thought that way. Notice how just the simple act of changing your vision begins to soften your resistance and bring you closer to contentment.

- Start a daily gratitude practice. At dinner or on the drive to school or work, think of all the things that are good in your life.

- Pick a day for each person in your family or circle of friends to be the chooser of a shared activity. If it is not your day, practice being accepting of things, even if they are not exactly to your liking.

- Get into nature and notice the contentment that comes from sitting under a tree in the sunshine or listening to the soft sound of the breeze.

- Next time you are frustrated, hang in a forward bend and take ten deep, conscious breaths. Let attachment (Raga) and aversion (Dvesa) drain out. As you come up slowly, return with acceptance and contentment in your mind.

- When asked to do something, especially something that you do not want to do, try doing it with a cheerful attitude and offering *more* than is requested.

QUESTIONS FOR FURTHER REFLECTION

Take a moment with your journal now to answer the following questions. Or find a quiet pause sometime today to remember the quality of contentment and contemplate these thoughts further.

- Notice how much energy you have in the past, the present, and the future. If you were to bring your full attention into the now, without any preconceptions or expectations, how would you feel?

- Notice when you feel ultra-reactive. How can practicing contentment diffuse reactivity?

- Notice when you are being judgmental. Switch into a more accepting attitude. How does practicing acceptance make you feel free?

- Think of a situation where you want something to happen. Check your expectations. Are they realistic? Does the other person see them as realistic? If you let go of some of them, would you feel more relaxed?

- How does your body feel when you are attached to something going your way? How does your body feel when you are open to whatever happens?

- Consider how your thoughts make you feel upset or content. How could you choose peace and contentment in your thoughts about yourself and others? Write or say a few of your contented thoughts.

AFFIRMATIONS TO POST AND REMEMBER

Affirmations solidify beliefs in our subconscious minds, creating a foundation from which we can then manifest positive change in our outer lives. Repeat these often with strong intensity and full faith.

- I accept where and how I am right now. Everything is temporary and I choose to be content now.

- I can relax in this moment. Nothing needs to change for me to *choose* to relax.

- I accept my imperfection and the imperfection of life.

- I use each experience that comes my way as an opportunity for growth and learning how to love more completely.

- I choose peace and contentment no matter what.

Chapter Eight

....

Right Action (Tapas): Pairing Passion and Non-Attachment

Right and fervent actions
facilitate mastery over the senses
and reveal the true Self within.
Sutra ii.43

To create the happy life we dream of, a combination of passionate engagement and disciplined living is necessary. The purpose of right action (Tapas) is to keep us on the pathway toward *true* happiness rather than allowing ourselves to be pulled impulsively toward short-lived pleasures. Finding our balance through sincere effort, physically and mentally, this Sutra assures us that we will awaken an inspired consciousness and find joy in sharing our unique gifts with the world.

Tapas, along with the next two Niyamas on Self-reflection (Swadhaya) and devotion (Iswara Pranidhana,) make up what is referred to as the yoga of action or kriya yoga. Will-fueled effort is applied to transform any mental or physical obstacles that plague us, such as apathy, laziness, distraction, or narcissism. By employing temporary restraints like fasting, holding silence, or regulating our breath, we weave the practice of purification into daily life. Through these spiritual practices (sadhana), we enhance the expression of our natural brilliance, creativity, and joy.

In order to facilitate this inner clarification, Tapas practice must be understood in the same way as the use of physical fire. We need self-control for right action the way fire needs to be controlled for right use. A contained fire is helpful for heating or cooking, but a wildfire is destructive. Tapas, as a cleansing fire within us, helps us achieve clearer and higher consciousness. But too much effort based in the ego's need for achievement or validation destroys our spiritual progress.

Willpower versus Willfulness

In order to cultivate Tapas, we need willpower. Not desire or intention, but an unbreakable will that generates force and action. Desires or intentions without will force are nothing but impotent wishes. Will, on the other hand, creates energy and requires that we employ it in constructive, focused ways. It is the link between positive thought and actual manifestation.

Will is the essential component for success in any endeavor, and, like any muscle, the more we use it, the larger it grows. It is stimulated by enthusiasm, a cheerful attitude, determination, and love. Willpower is fueled by attunement to our inner wisdom and sustained by it as we apply concentration and continuity to our chosen course.

Will is an instrument of change and the greater our will force, the greater the change we can effect, both internally and externally. By consciously using willpower to burn through personal obstacles and tap the unlimited Source of life energy, this Sutra describes how we are freed from physical and mental limitations.

There is, however, a difference between applying the power of will to a challenging situation and pushing through that experience with willfulness. The former is the sincere discipline required for success. The latter is the ego serving its own desire. The first way enlivens us. The second exhausts us. Like any other yogic practice, the effort of purifying action (Tapas) must be combined with reflection, discernment, and non-attachment for best results. In this way, we can see where our motivation and action falls on the spectrum of willfulness to willpower.

Through Tapas practice, we learn to apply just the right amount of effort or discipline to all aspects of life. By exchanging ego-based willfulness for soul-centered willpower, we engage with our activities and relationships easefully. We also release ourselves from the roller coaster of the ego's pride in success and suffering from failure. Spirit empowers our will when it is guided by soul-centered wisdom and a desire to serve the good of all beings, and enables us to accomplish without limits.

Tapas and Dharma

What we are meant to accomplish is determined by our soul's purpose (dharma) for this lifetime. This is our unique contribution to the world and is usually perceived as we combine what we love and feel most passionately about with service to the greater good of all beings. Our enthusiasm is the fire that burns away any blocks within, such as fear or doubt. To fully express our dharma or unique soul purpose, we must stoke that fire strongly but keep it under wise control. In this way, it can fuel the accomplishment of our goals without burning us out or leaving us stifled through lack of tending.

Our dharma gives us focus, a charge to action, and a gauge to know when we stray from what is important. By knowing our purpose, we have a guide by which to determine the validity of all our choices. For example, if running an honest and stress-free business is part of our dharma, then anything that compromises our integrity or ability to feel peaceful is not a good choice. Knowing what the overall goal is, we make clear decisions in how and where we expend effort and will on a daily basis.

Take a moment to consider what your dharma is and how your life at this time aligns, or not, with this purpose. Whether or not this is clear to you at this time, Tapas practice purifies us, removing that which stands in our way of full expression, such as negative thinking or bad habits. If we are prepared to do our clarifying work, applying right effort and at the same time holding non-attachment to the results of our actions, we assure that the ego is not being served but rather being placed *in service to* the soul.

In future chapters, other limbs outline practices that purify and discipline the body and mind, like right posture (Asana), life energy control (Pranayama), and deep concentration (Dharana). All of these clear away impurities of the ego, revealing in its place our true nature, the inner light of the soul. In order to be fully alive, we must be on fire with purpose, and use our will to move forward with undaunted determination toward our goals. By bringing passion, diligence, and devotion, coupled with non-attachment, to each day, our unique soul purpose will be revealed. Then life will be a grand adventure, enjoyed even when difficult.

Tapas of Thought

There are three main categories in which Tapas practice is accomplished: thought, speech, and action. Since thought is the powerful initiator of creation, we begin here. All that is now manifest was originally a thought in the Universal Consciousness and our minds are a part of the Great Mind. We have access to infinite intelligence. So if we want to create or change anything, we must begin in thought.

As we have already noted, however, habituated patterns of thought can subtly sabotage our progress, even if we know our desired direction in life. The uncontrolled thoughts of the fidgety, egocentric, self-serving mind are the demise of many intelligent people and must be tamed. In Tapas we continue watching the content of our thoughts in order to consciously direct them in a positive way to create the life we wish for. All the practices of the Eight Limbs help to purify the restless mind, especially the later branches of interiorization (Pratyahara) and concentration (Dharana). Practicing Tapas in regard to thought is the preliminary step to these deeper practices.

Repetitive thought creates neural pathways called Samskaras in the yogic teachings. Like driving with the emergency brake on in our car, negative Samskaras that result from difficult experiences or Karma impede our efforts at self-improvement and wreak havoc on the accomplishment of our goals. So we begin by astutely watching our thoughts, bringing them into the light of awareness. We cleanse the mind by catching and discarding judgments, fears, self-doubts, and limitations, as these disrupt our will force.

Once we can catch these detrimental thought patterns, then we can replace them with their positive opposite, a practice the Yoga Sutras call Pratipaksha Bhavana. Tapas of thought uses this simple technique to escort out all mental saboteurs. Simply replace any negative thought with its positive opposite. Even chronic pessimists can change through this simple yet profound practice, one thought at a time.

Like a movie producer who films the same scene from close up and then from a wide angle, we can step out of the personal attachment (Raga) or aversion (Dvesa) to the experience at hand and watch what is occurring with objectivity. This further development of mindfulness or witness consciousness enables us to observe thought, feeling, and experience, rather than be immersed in it. It is the key to shifting from the perspective of the ego (i.e., "I, me, mine") to the Self (all as one).

We change our lives by utilizing willpower to redirect habituated patterns of thought that drive behaviors that keep us suffering. Setbacks then become temporary learning opportunities rather than permanent failures and we assign personal meaning to crisis and challenge. In all these ways, ordinary moments lead us to spiritual awakening.

Tapas of Speech

As a reflection and extension of our thoughts, our speech also requires the purification practice of Tapas. Granted, we all need to speak our minds, but not everything that comes to mind needs saying! We should regulate the outflow of thought by pausing for internal reflection before speaking. Exercising self-control, we can ask ourselves, "Is what I am about to say uplifting? Is it loving and compassionate? Is it true? Is it relevant and necessary?" These integrate the practices of Ahimsa and Satya, and help to keep our speech pure. Speaking unkindly or reactively devitalizes our will and demagnetizes our Life Force Energy.

Additionally, our vocal quality affects how others receive us, and the information we wish to convey. If we speak harshly and loudly, people may withdraw and reject what we have to say. If we mumble or fib, people may not trust us. Bringing clear intention to our tone and to our words is practicing Tapas and creates more effective communication. Additionally, we can combine Tapas and Santosha by being content *not* speaking at times.

Tapas of Action

In the realm of physical actions, in order to transform obstacles, we start by identifying where the imbalance lies. Looking back to Brahmacharya, we check how our energy level is in relation to our physical activities. If it is low, maybe an adjustment in our exercise or food intake is needed. A purifying action could be a fast or cleanse to remove toxins from the body, allowing the organs to rest and revitalize. If our energy level is racing and anxious, we can apply energy-control techniques (Pranayama) discussed in chapter twelve in order to come back into balance.

Maybe we spend too much time looking at social media or television, or we stay too long at the office and forgo healthy activity. Are we draining energy and will force through over-stimulation of the senses, overwork, or laziness? By bringing full attention to each moment, we can more accurately address what is out of balance.

Happiness lies in being able to master our urges, impulses, and reactions. Choosing positive, ethical, supportive environments and friends enables us to be stronger in our healthy choices. We are not free if habits of thought, speech, or action dictate our choices. Recognizing where we are enslaved by our habits is the first step toward breaking those patterns of behavior that do not serve our dharma purpose.

The Terrible Nature of Habit

Every time we repeat an action or a thought, we create impressions on the consciousness. These mental blueprints, the Samskaras, become grooves in the physiological brain. Habitual actions and the accompanying thought patterns become so ingrained that when even the slightest attention is placed there, or we come near the action, we are ensnared again and the grooves are cut deeper. When in the grip of a habit, we are afraid to change and eventually the ruts become so deep that monumental effort is required to literally get "out of the groove." The influence of bad habits of thought or behavior make us prefer little fleeting moments of pleasure to the joy of true right action. They seem to satisfy but inevitably disappoint, creating satiation without satisfaction and the soul goes on seeking its eternal happiness.

Willpower is required to do what we know is right and good and to avoid what we know is not healthy or positive. By using the Tapas practice of will force, we can eradicate happiness-killing habits. Make up your mind and do it! Will the habit to leave and feel the spiritual power that kicks in when attention is clear and focused.

Breaking the shackles of habit requires intensity, earnestness, and devotion. We can start with one small thing to change and stick to it until we have erased the habit of thought or action. In this way, we train our mind's power of command and its capacity to change anything we choose. Then we can move on to larger endeavors and liberate ourselves from the terrible grip of habitual behavior.

Perseverance through Challenging Times

Consistent training of thought, word, and action is required to become a true yogi. It is one thing to feel a flare of passion, but it is another to feed that flame and keep it on course. This is the discipline of Tapas.

The trials of life come to teach us to keep a calm mind and a persevering will, thereby becoming stronger and clearer as a result. In the same way an athlete in training improves by competing with more skilled opponents, challenges stimulate us to greater heights of wisdom and of love. When we choose happiness under all conditions and give kindness to all who cross our path, regardless of what they give us, we open the door to joy. Each small movement in this direction strengthens us. We can trust that whatever our particular environment or circumstances, it is perfect for our spiritual growth.

Proper use of self-control, will force, and the elimination of doubt secures our progress. The more we practice and stay the course, the more inner help and resources appear, awakened from within the Divine subconscious that lights our discriminatory faculties. As our will is aligned with soul wisdom, faith becomes our traveling companion. We cultivate the habit of inwardly conversing with Spirit, releasing our ego-based control of things to the highest good for all involved. We concentrate on gratitude for what we have been given rather than what we miss. Eventually, we surrender the ego fully in recognition that Spirit is the ultimate doer of all actions and the One to whom all results are due. As the *Bhagavad Gita* directs, we perform all actions undisturbed by their results, immersed in the thought of the Divine, forsaking attachment.

Through the conscious action of passionate perseverance and non-attachment, we put ourselves in harmony with Universal Goodness. As we decide time and again to be happy and to live life to the fullest, no matter what, we enjoy a trust in the cosmic order that is larger than our mind's comprehension. This mental evenness during all states of activities is yoga. And yoga is liberation.

DAILY PRACTICES

Integrate an active practice of right and fervent action into your daily life. Look for the ways in which you get blocked mentally or physically and apply strong-willed effort to clear your way forward.

- To build willpower, follow these steps. Choose something you have not done before and determine wholeheartedly to do it. Make a simple, reasonable goal and concentrate completely. Refuse to consider failure.

- Next time you feel angry and want to shout, regulate your voice to speak softly and notice the difference you feel as a result.

- Watch for habitual behaviors or reactions. Practicing Tapas of action and speech, choose a different route.

- Practice Tapas of thought by repeating an affirmation or mantra to focus the mind and to direct more will into the desired outcome.

- Spend some more time identifying your dharma, or soul purpose, the way in which your uniqueness benefits the good of all. Consider any needed changes in your daily actions or thoughts to support that purpose and life goal.

Questions for Further Reflection

Take a moment with your journal now to answer the following questions. Or find a quiet pause sometime today to remember the practice of right effort and contemplate these thoughts further.

- Assess your Tapas level at this time through the following questions. On a daily basis, doing whatever you are doing, do you feel restless, bored, lazy, unambitious, or exhausted? Or do you feel inspired, charged with energy, focused and excited to give something of yourself to the world?

- If you need to ignite your inner flame, spark it up with these reflections. What invigorates you? What always comes to mind when you think about what you want to do? What are you really good at and how could that help others?

- Do you avoid challenging situations, conflict in relationships, or difficult emotions inside? If so, practice Tapas by stepping closer to the fire consciously and compassionately.

- Do you over-exert and experience burnout and frustration? How can you apply the principle of right effort for greater ease?

- What mental saboteurs do you need to counteract by replacing them with a positive thought?

AFFIRMATIONS TO POST AND REMEMBER

Affirmations solidify beliefs in our subconscious minds, creating a foundation from which we can then manifest positive change in our outer lives. Repeat these often with strong intensity and full faith.

- My will is aligned with my soul's wisdom.

- Through my willingness, I find the way.

- I align with right effort (Tapas). I feel balanced and at ease, passionate yet non-attached.

- I show up fully to all life has to offer me today. By practicing courageous willingness, I become stronger and braver each day.

- Aligned with my dharma, I lovingly live and share my skills and passions for the good of all beings.

Chapter Nine

....

Self-Reflection
(Swadhaya): Discovering
Your True Nature

Through study of sacred texts
and introspection one communes
with the Divine Self.
Sutra ii.44

To know oneself is a humbling undertaking. People spend years
in therapy analyzing themselves and trying to understand why
they are the way they are. By observing our beliefs, behaviors,
and choices with objectivity, we discover whether or not they
are life-affirming It is important to take responsibility for our
personal history and our actions, as well as our habits, fears, and
doubts. Hopefully we can do all of this with some measure of
humor and without judgment. By refusing to hide from what

is within, we prepare the way for the deeper levels of introspection and awareness that the Sutra on Swadhaya teaches.

The Yoga Sutras speak of the Universal Self, as designated with a capital "S," being manifest in infinite ways as the unique personalities we call self, which is labeled with a small "s." This Sutra on Swadhaya encourages introspection on both the small self and the Divine Self, particularly through the study of sacred texts. Swadhaya is the second in the trio of Niyamas that comprise the yoga of action (kriya yoga). It inspires reflection on who we are and why we are here, so we may feel the joyful integration of our individual attributes with our expansive nature as part of Universal Consciousness.

To shift in the direction of identifying with the Supreme Self rather than with the individual self, we must blend the honest witnessing of our human challenges with the surrender of all negative self-concepts. When we see ourselves as a unique part of the Divine Creation, we realize our *innate* worth and goodness, whether or not we have received a sense of value from our human families or personal successes. Analysis of our human imperfections is not meant to be discouraging, but rather an entryway to finding the road home to our Soul nature.

We can reach a state of peace if we combine the honest self-assessment process of psychotherapy with the direct perception of our true nature as spiritual beings. If we miss this key component and overwork self-analysis without an expanded perception of Self, then therapy can actually become a distraction, encouraging identification with the wrong aspects of our being.

Outside In or Inside Out

Most humans have a deep, innate desire to *know* who they are and why they are here. As we will see in chapter eleven on Asana practice, there are two directions we can take to study the Self. Practice of right posture (Asana) is the vehicle that many Western practitioners are attracted to initially to journey from outside in, through the development of the body and its subtle expressions of the Soul. They are often surprised by the inner transformation that awakens as a result of physical rebalancing. Others are compelled to understand yogic philosophy first and then find their way to the value of physical practices that support the inner journey. Either way requires time, focus, and energy, and eventually both ways bring us within.

Moving inward where awareness of Self enables us to know what is right for us gives us surety as we navigate the complexities of human life. By learning to listen to our Self, we clear the cobwebs of self-doubt and fear, hallmarks of our ego nature, and we open to the voice of the soul. This ignites intuition.

Intuition is our soul's messenger, an inner guide to the best answers for life's challenges. The voice of the intuition is distinctly different from the voice of the ego. It is a humble, persistent, consistent call to goodness and love. It is available to us all but first we must cultivate the ability to hear and heed it. For some, intuitive messaging comes as a combination of thinking and feeling, guiding them toward what is right. Others may have a more kinesthetic sensation centered in the region of the heart that lets them know they are on the right track.

To be sure, what we are hearing is the soul talking and not our ego, we start by noticing when our mind, heart, and body coordinate in total awareness and all our senses are in harmony. When we feel no conflict within, no emotional triggers or agendas, just peace and security, then we are hearing the inner guide of wisdom.

The second way to know is when we have the objectivity to separate the form of the need from the essence of the need. For example, our child is not doing well in school. The essence of the need is for him to do better. The form may take many different shapes, such as private tutoring, extra help from us, or possibly a change of schools. If we can let go of the mental anguish over what we think *should* be, the right way will become clear. When we let go of attachment to what resolution will look like, we feel no pressure or tension, but rather, a calm knowing that the appropriate form will manifest to fulfill the essence of the need.

The third way of knowing our inner guidance is on track is through a list of three questions that can serve as a test until we are comfortable trusting our inner voice. Although these initially rely on some analysis, eventually we develop a sense of direct knowing that transcends the mental process. If the answers to the following questions are yes, trust that decision.

- Is it legal, moral, and healthy for everyone involved?

- Does it preserve the dignity and well-being of everyone involved?

- Does it increase the love and compassion in my heart?

Not Knowing

There will be times when we receive no answers from within. No one likes to feel unsure, powerless, or out of control, but if we are living in alignment with truth (Satya) and have honestly done our work to silently know intuition's answer and still sense no clear way to proceed, then we can rest in not knowing. We can practice contentment (Santosha), trusting that although it may not be the time for us to know the answer to a particular question or challenge, overall we are in our right place and our right place right now is in not knowing. This can be peaceful, especially if we have faith that when the time is right to move forward we will know which direction to go.

This is the perfect time to dig into the study of the Higher Self through sacred texts as suggested by the Sutra on Swadhaya. By reflecting upon the universal truth they hold, we educate ourselves on our own expansive nature, the Divine Self within. And through this, we are guided to a greater understanding of our human self as its reflection. The more dedicated our study, the more we understand our strengths and weaknesses and the more freedom we have in utilizing our strong points and overcoming the weak ones. As a result of this revealed wisdom, we build greater intuitive faculties and live with more intention and purpose.

Definition of a Sacred Text

Any scripture that has been divinely or supernaturally revealed or inspired, such as the *Vedas*, the *Bible*, the *I Ching*, or the Yoga

Sutras is a sacred text. These manuscripts stimulate a desire for inward realization and reveal truth in ever-deeper layers depending on our consciousness at the time we read them.

Initially it is valuable to compare several translations of whichever sacred text we feel compelled to study to find the one that speaks to us naturally, like a beloved teacher. With our chosen material, we should select just one passage or teaching to contemplate and embody for a week or more. It does no good to read a passage, be inspired for a moment or two, and then forget it. The goal is to live and breathe it before moving on to the next. Intellectual comprehension of the ancient revelations is not enough. They must be realized within. If not, vanity, false ego satisfaction, and undigested knowledge will result. Remembering the Niyama of purity (Saucha) is essential so that we do not continually seek new doctrines that will in effect lead us to spiritual starvation or indigestion if not assimilated and put into practice.

To accurately study sacred texts, we need to utilize intuition for a more complete understanding than what the limited intellect can deliver. The doors of true perception rarely open just with the mind. Deepest knowing of Self arrives through intuitive personal experience and empirical evidence based on inner practices that require spiritual discipline and enthusiasm. Through an intuitive approach, we feel the inherent truth in many outer expressions of faith, religion, and philosophy.

Truth found in any sacred scripture produces results in accordance with its proper use in life. Like a mathematic equation, the principles have to be applied. There is absolutely no comparison between reading a truth and actually absorbing it and making it our own through communion with Self.

The best time for reflective study is after meditation when our intuitive awareness is heightened. This is when we can see beyond the veil of limited human self to infinite Supreme Self, which the Sutras describe as being ever present, ever conscious, and ever joyous. It is only because most of the time we are looking through the vehicle of small self that we think we are separate beings defined by our personalities and roles in this particular life. A magnificent new paradigm opens when we stop identifying ourselves as someone's mother, father, wife, or husband and start knowing ourselves as complete, radiant souls made of love and light. This Self knowing enables us to do whatever we do with creativity and freedom.

The perspective of Patanjali's Sutras is that the Divine Self is within all things. The Eight Limbs of Yoga give us the perfect combination of practices to move beyond our basic comprehension of self as our human persona. In the last chapter we learned the value of being mindful of our thought, speech, and action (Tapas) in an effort to evolve our consciousness. As we progress on with upcoming limbs we will see how the use of right posture (Asana) liberates the flow of energy in the body, preparing us for the discipline of interiorization of consciousness (Pratyahara). Eventually this enables us to enter the stillness of meditation (Dhyana), wherein we perceive Divinity expressing itself through our unique lives.

Art of Introspection

As we gain initial glimmers of the Divine Self that is within us, we can then circle back to assessing ways of improving our human self. The most productive way to introspect is through daily watchfulness of the strategies the ego employs to shield itself from exposure.

Starting with our thoughts, we notice what consciousness is predominant. If it is pessimistic or overly centered on self rather than others, it is time to employ the will force of Tapas to honestly and objectively root out what lies in our way. We take action by mentally replacing the thought or quality that is disturbing us, such as fear, with the opposite quality we wish to cultivate, such as courage. This transformation of thought by cultivating the opposite thought (Pratipaksha Bhavana) lightens our load as we practice putting the ego in service to the Self.

By applying the quality we want to cultivate in both little and big ways in daily life, change happens subtly. We can utilize the selected teaching or quality in multiple ways at home, at work, everywhere throughout the day. For example, if reactive anger is an issue, we can apply the quality of patience by slowing down and being more thoughtful before responding. One day we will notice this has become the norm. Other people's reactions to us will be our gauge. Those who know us help us see our blind spots more clearly.

At the end of each day, we can analyze how well we did, using the Yamas and Niyamas as our guide. Did we give in to moods or did we cheerfully practice Santosha? Were we peaceful and truthful in our communications, practicing Ahimsa and Satya? Did we apply a balanced amount of energy and effort to work, exercise, creative pursuits, and spiritual practice, reflecting Brahmacharya and Tapas? Did we seek ways to serve others, offering Astheya and Aparigraha?

Return to Love

The process of attunement to Self requires that we use the practices of the Eight Limbs to continuously reorient toward who we really are. We must keep in mind our innate value as expressions of the Divine Self, which is magnificent, infinitely creative, loving, and beautiful. Then we can navigate our human journey with all of its ups and downs easefully and effect positive change in the world through our unique attributes and skills. If we were not validated as children in our worth and goodness, now is the time to choose a different perspective, one that is self-honoring and anchored in spiritual Self love. This shift in identification is the most essential inner change we can make.

The practice of Swadhaya breaks through the aspects of self that keep us limited and fearful. When we recognize that all the qualities we so easily admire in others—like courage, strength, or creativity—are within ourselves, we see through the *real eyes* of love. We *realize* ourselves as sacred, spiritual beings, deserving of all goodness. We extend love to all of those around us and we feel it return to us in increasing measure.

Divinity is within and Self-reflection (Swadhaya) brings it into clear focus, revealing our purpose for being. From this place of Self-understanding and purpose, we open to life from a dynamic place of centeredness and joy.

Daily Practice

Integrate an active practice of reflection into your daily life. Check in with both your authentic individual self and your transcendent spiritual Self and notice how and when each one is present and active in your day.

- Carve out quiet time every day. Commute to school or work in silence or take a quiet walk at lunch so you can be with your own thoughts and listen to your intuition.

- Lose the background noise in the house. Turn off televisions, iPods, cell phones, and computers. Listen within instead.

- Practice solitude often. Check in with your intuition for deep wisdom on right choices and actions.

- Write a personal mission statement. Make it an affirmation of who you wish to be in the world, a reflection of your personal purpose and meaning.

- Every evening, spend a few moments reflecting upon the day and the consciousness with which you lived it.

- Read a variety of sacred texts, like the *Upanishads*, *Bhagavad Gita*, *Bible*, *Tao Te Ching*, or translations of the Yoga Sutras until you find one that really resonates in your heart, then dig deep into the study of that one. Reflect on what it makes you think and feel.

Questions for Further Reflection

Take a moment with your journal now to answer the following questions. Or find a quiet pause sometime today to remember the necessity for Self-reflection and contemplate these thoughts further.

- Use everything and everyone as a mirror through which you discover something about yourself. Ask yourself, "How does the quality I appreciate or dislike in another reflect an aspect of my own self?"

- If you really knew that you and everyone around you were part of the one Divine Self, how would you behave differently? How would you treat yourself? Others?

- If you knew that your smallest actions influenced the entire rest of the world, what kind of mindfulness would you adopt?

- How can you shine your unique light more brightly? How does the Divine Self want to manifest through you today?

Affirmations to Post and Remember

Affirmations solidify beliefs in our subconscious minds, creating a foundation from which we can then manifest positive change in our outer lives. Repeat these often with strong intensity and full faith.

- I am worthy of life, love, joy, and happiness.

- My true Self is perfect, happy, and free.

- When my light and joy are challenged, I reflect and learn what is necessary and then shine even brighter.

- I choose a consciousness of love today.

- I honor myself and all beings as part of the Supreme Self.

Chapter Ten

••••••••••••••••••••••

Devotion
(Iswara Pranidhana):
Surrendering to Love

Absolute devotion and surrender
to the Divine enables soul freedom.
Sutra ii.45

In different translations of the Sutras, various names are given to the Divine. This essence is called Iswara, the Light Within, Supreme Self, Universal Consciousness, Divine Light, Divine Consciousness, and Divine Self. We can call it Inspiration, Source, God, Spirit, Oneness, Creative Force, or Love. The Divine is both manifest in all things material and unmanifest as pure Consciousness. Ultimately, it does not matter what we choose to call it. What matters is that we become so immersed *in* it that we know ourselves *as* it. Our love simply becomes Love.

Our light simply becomes Light. And our dedication becomes wholehearted devotion by recognizing the sacred in all that is within and around us.

Devotion (Iswara Pranidhana) is the key, according to this Sutra, to unlocking the greatest levels of love within us. By surrendering the identification with our small self in complete devotion to our highest Self, we find ultimate happiness. Our hearts are transformed when the mind and the ego step out of the way and when we offer up self-consciousness and personal agenda in service to the Divine. When we attune to the energy of love and walk through the world seeing everything and everyone as part of the One, we experience unparalleled levels of well-being and joy. The trio of Tapas (right action), Swadhaya (reflection on Self), and Iswara Pranidhana (wholehearted devotion) form the transformative combination of yoga in action called kriya yoga.

Devotion versus Discipline

Although discipline and commitment are necessary for all spiritual practice, discipline alone can become cold and routine when not coupled with devotion or dedication. We are dedicated to the people and things we love. Devotion holds the vital element of love, which makes it more sustainable than discipline for most people. It takes the form of focused attention, so it is important to be intentional about what we choose both outwardly and inwardly, because whatever we devote our time and energy to determines the course of our life. In order to feel true bliss and joy, this Sutra says our devotion (Iswara Pranidhana) must be to an aspect of the Divine that brings us closer to love.

The ancient yogis, coming from the Vedic perspective that Universal Consciousness cannot be quantified by any one definition or image, sought a personal experience of Divinity. It is valuable for us to assess where our familial or religious concepts may be hindering rather than helping our experience of the Essence within. As we approach the deeper inner practices of the Eight Limbs, we must be willing to have a wholly new interchange with our Spiritual Self.

If we do not currently have a personal sense of the Divine, it is helpful to consider the type or form of love we most desire. For some that may be a nurturing, protecting love. For others it may be a creative, inspiring love. Everyone has a love they feel is absolutely needed and essential. This is the aspect of the Divine to call out to. This is the portal through which we can cultivate devotion. Be so in love with it that nothing else matters and ask in a simple heartfelt prayer that the Divine reveal itself in this way.

Love as Spiritual Practice (Sadhana)

According to this Sutra, Iswara Pranidhana is the practice of devotion with the courage, conviction, and dedication of our *whole heart.* Usually we reserve a bit of our heart's love in self-protection, but to practice this teaching we must drop our ego-centric agenda of getting love personally and lose ourselves in the universal energy of Love. By doing this, we set ourselves up for an experience that is bigger than our individual understanding or expression of love. The moment we feel ourselves opening into transcendent, non-personalized love, we realize it is many times greater than any human occurrence of loving.

If we monitor the predominant consciousness we operate from on a daily basis, we will see when it is one of fear or one of love. The consciousness of fear takes us further away from Source. Love brings us closer. To remember our infinite nature *as* Love, and to become unconditionally loving, is of utmost importance for our lasting happiness and fulfillment in life.

Through introspection (Swadhaya), we notice when our consciousness falls into patterns that prevent our evolution in this regard. The predominant obstacles named by the Sutras are egocentricity, attachment, aversion, ignorance, fear, illness, lethargy, impatience, doubt, resignation, distraction, arrogance, and loss of confidence.

Any of these states of consciousness impedes our personal development and separate us from love. When we keep calm and approach daily trials as training to become stronger in our ability to give and receive love, then we are rewarded with greater faith. We do not need to pray for obstacles to be removed but rather for the strength to overcome them. In this way, our devotion and our love get immeasurably stronger.

Intentional loving as spiritual practice (sadhana) requires that we acknowledge the shared Divinity between all beings. Any limitation we feel in loving others is usually because we are relating to them as their ego or small self, through our ego or small self, rather than through our unified Divine nature. By shifting our perspective to see others and ourselves as souls within human forms, it becomes easier to be dedicated to love, no matter what is happening between us.

We release anger more easily. We spend less time fighting for our way. We forgive with ease and we meet people with empathy and understanding, even if they are not giving us what we desire in the moment. We keep our hearts open no matter what and practice peacefulness (Ahimsa) and generosity (Astheya) when we are confronted with challenging personal circumstances.

Additionally, we can reflect upon our human relationships as mirrors of our current relationship with Spirit. Meaning that if we feel a lack of trust in our intimate relationships, we will probably see the same pattern in how we feel about the Divine. If we feel a lack of time and attention from our loved ones, we can reflect on how much time and attention we are giving to our primary relationship with Source.

What Is Required

Besides being willing to self-reflect, within the practice of devotion, an offering is required. Paramahansa Yogananda, who is known for bringing the teachings of Kriya Yoga to the West and for his spiritual classic *Autobiography of a Yogi*,[10] calls the surrender of self the greatest devotional offering we can make. To lay down our small self or ego in loving service to the great Divine Self is a life-changing sacrifice. Fortunately, due to the circular nature of devotion and love, the more devotion we practice, the more love we feel, and the more love we feel, the more devotion we want to practice. When we can acknowledge Source as

---

10   Paramahansa Yogananda, *Autobiography of a Yogi* (Los Angeles: Self Realization Fellowship, 1998).

the ultimate Doer, Creator, and Lover of all, then we can dedicate the fruits of all our accomplishments to Spirit. In this way, we cultivate humility and connection. And when we release the desire to receive benefit from our actions, ultimate happiness comes as our grace-filled reward.

This level of surrender and offering requires intense trust. The ego is not keen on relinquishing its position of power in our lives. In order for this to happen, we must know the Self to which we are dedicating our love and trust. Sri Patanjali encourages us to look beyond the temporary and limited human experience to know our self as part and parcel of the great Cosmic Self. In so doing, the need to protect and defend the needs of a separate self fade away and devotion is no longer to something outside but rather to the One within.

In Our Stillness, the Divine's Silence Ceases

To personally experience the loving Awareness that upholds the Universe within ourselves, we need silence. But how can we find silence in this world that is full of noise and activity? Breaking news, rapid-fire entertainment, and ceaseless social media flood our lives. If we spend each day filling our brains with information from the outside, without balancing this with an inner connection to tranquility, we will never tap into the wealth of true wisdom that lives within.

The only way to develop stronger connection to the voice of the True Self that guides from within is to calm the restless body and mind, and to silence the voice of the screaming ego.

Divine guidance is built into all humans through the instruments of conscience and intuition. Conscience is its first level and intuition is its more developed counterpart. If we are overly emotional, anxious, or analytical, these cannot be heard. Like any muscle that strengthens with gradual exercise, employing the practices that lie ahead in the Eight Limbs strengthens our intuitive sixth sense.

This requires a willingness to overcome the fear of stillness and what we might find within, as discussed in the previous chapter on Self-reflection (Swadhaya). Rumi, the thirteenth-century Sufi poet and mystic who often wrote about the spiritual journey, said that silence is the language of God. Truth is found in silence. Inspiration, understanding, rest, renewal, healing, and peace all emanate from silence. The ability to transcend whatever keeps us blocked or limited is found in silence through the still, small voice of guidance sourced in Love.

Creating Silence

To develop a relationship with silence, we need to blend the committed energy of discipline with the loving energy of devotion. Through discipline we maintain our practices, accomplish goals, and meet deadlines. Through devotion we renew our daily willingness to show up. Over time, if not practiced together, many people rebel against discipline that is not enhanced with love.

First, we commit to outer silence by intentionally carving out quiet time each day, no matter what. It could be 5:00 a.m. at home, 11:00 a.m. at the office, or noon in the car. We can start with five minutes a day and be dedicated to it. As we become comfortable with silence, it acts as a soothing balm to the incessant noise of life.

We create inner silence by gently greeting the flood of thoughts, emotions, adrenaline, and anxiety that arrives when we get quiet outwardly. We do not need to judge the layers of feelings, frustrations, sorrows, rage, tension, and the million notes to self. Silence is patient. Just be present. Eventually the mind stops thrashing about and we enter a blissful moment of inner stillness, feel the pulse of intuition, and realize that inspiration, renewal, and peace are always within reach.

Using Silence Constructively

The practice of silence for peace of mind and attunement to highest wisdom can also be shared with others who are struggling. By holding a kind, empathetic silence rather than trying to fix the problem or person, we give a love that is deeper than words. If we offer uninterrupted listening, we honor the other person's process and feelings. Although we may not always agree, we can be present with respect and the willingness to understand.

To do this, we must relax, surrender our personal agenda, and recognize that we are all a part of the Divine Oneness. If we find ourselves moving into impatience or judgment, we can employ self-control (Brahmacharya), silently think of that person's good qualities, or politely end the time together in order to reflect on why we feel triggered. Loving silence enables all involved to listen to their intuitive guidance before continuing.

In this potent stillness, hearts open and we return to our practice of dedication to Source with no expectation of personal return.

In the spaciousness of silence combined with devotion, we cultivate an abiding relationship with our Highest Self through intuitive wisdom, and we find the anchor of love and peace that enables our lives to unfold with ease.

Prayer

In chapters fourteen and fifteen, we will explore the devotional practices of concentration (Dharana) and meditation (Dhyana), which are similar to the uninterrupted listening described above, in which we commune with the Divine in stillness. Prayer is a complimentary devotional practice in which we contact the Divine through loving communication. Prayer can take many forms and should emanate from our hearts through the language of our souls. If our heart is dedicated to the sacred within and around us, we can pray with words or without them. We can pray to surrender the ego and stand in awe of the mystery of Life (Iswara). We can pray for positive change for ourselves and for the world. We can pray to be led inward to an awareness of true Self or for the ability to be devoted to what is highest and most loving. We can pray with gratitude until all that exists within us is Love and a faith that is beyond understanding.

To withdraw our awareness from all objects of distraction, completely absorbing ourselves in one-pointed prayer and dedication takes us to profound peace and ever-renewing bliss. Through this and other practices that support wholehearted devotion, we will know Self as unending Love and Joy.

DAILY PRACTICE

Integrate an active practice of devotion into your daily life. Allow a gentle redefinition of the Divine to present itself to you and begin releasing attachment to the ego.

- Dedicate everything you do today to the Divine or to Love. Offer all actions and results to the highest good for all involved.

- Listen to the quiet voices of guidance that come in silence to lead you on your path.

- Listen to someone with your heart. Try to filter out the tone or attitude and just receive the information they are imparting. Then look behind the words for what they are feeling.

- Notice where your choices, decisions, and actions come from. Is it a consciousness of fear or love? Act only when you can identify love as the motivating force.

- Make a simple altar in your house with special items that represent the Divine that you are devoted to.

QUESTIONS FOR FURTHER REFLECTION

Take a moment with your journal now to answer the following questions. Or find a quiet pause sometime today to remember the practice of devotion and contemplate these thoughts further.

- Can you feel the difference when someone is listening to you with her heart as well as her ears? How does it feel to listen to someone in this way?

- How do you employ discipline in your life? Would using devotion instead feel different?

- Why is the inner practice of devotion an important balance to outer yoga practice?

- How can you open into the mystery of the Divine?

- If something or someone has colored your perception of the Divine in a negative way, are you willing to drop that perspective and open to a new experience from within?

AFFIRMATIONS TO POST AND REMEMBER

Affirmations solidify beliefs in our subconscious minds, creating a foundation from which we can then manifest positive change in our outer lives. Repeat these often with strong intensity and full faith.

- In silence, I find my way to my heart.

- Where my devotion flows, my life follows.

- I am dedicated to the Divine within and without.

- I offer all that I do and all that I have back to Source.

- Devotion unlocks my heart and the pathway of my life unfolds.

PART THREE

....

Limbs Three–Eight

....

Deeper Practices:
Connecting
to Your
Divinity

Chapters eleven through sixteen cover limbs three through eight. These practices begin externally and gradually guide us to the most internalized states of being in which we access fully expanded awareness. Building on the solid groundwork of the Yamas and Niyamas, these actions and offerings take us to lasting happiness and liberation.

Beginning with the physical body, the Sutras address the practice of right posture (Asana) to create physical comfort and ease, eliminate restlessness, and prepare the body to be undistracted in meditation. Once the body is stable, the art of energy control (Pranayama) can be mastered. Pranayama regulates and enhances the subtle Life Force currents (prana) through which we move into subtler realms of awareness. Moving deeper within through sensory withdrawal (Pratyahara), we learn to detach the five senses from external stimuli and to develop a tranquil, receptive basis for meditation.

Once in stillness, the mind is controlled through concentrated focus (Dharana). We train ourselves to single-pointed attention for mental clarity and spiritual perception. With consistent practice of this, particularly in combination with devotion to Spirit within, we enter the state of meditation (Dhyana), a profound stillness in which consciousness flows uninterruptedly inward rather than outward.

When all remnants of personal ego are overcome and devotional focus is mastered, the bliss of reuniting individual consciousness with the universal One Consciousness is achieved. This is called Samadhi and is the culmination of the Eight Limbs of Yoga. All of these practices take time and dedicated effort. None can be rushed or skipped. A patient and peaceful approach assures our success and creates a happy life along the way.

Chapter Eleven

....

Right Posture (Asana): Physical Practice for Comfort and Ease

Right posture is steady and without strain.
By overcoming restlessness, through balanced effort and
focus on the Infinite within, one becomes undisturbed
by the fluctuating dualities of physical experience.
Sutras ii.46–ii.48

Asana is the practice of right posture to physically and energetically align the body, thereby creating ease and steadiness. Of the Eight Limbs, the physical practice of yoga postures is the one most familiar to people in the West. Cities across the United States are teeming with studios offering classes in Asana. And there is good reason. A healthy, tension-free body supports mental and emotional clarity and our ability to enter the stillness of meditation with greater comfort. Asana is also a vehicle for experiencing the Infinite Self within the finite self.

Yoga postures strengthen and stretch muscles, support structural alignment, stabilize joints, increase range of motion, build energy, release tension, rehabilitate injury, strengthen the immune system and organ function, alleviate pain, maintain youthfulness, and create a state of physical being that is both energized and relaxed. Some form of Asana practice is accessible to almost every body type and positive results are felt quickly, making it one of the most tangible of the Eight Limbs in its contribution to happiness through health and well-being.

Original Intent

The physical aspect of yoga, however, was never meant to be a stand-alone practice, or simply a form of exercise, as it has become today. And if undertaken without practicing the other limbs of inner reflection and transcendence, it can be counterproductive. Taken out of context, Asana may enhance the practitioner's identification with the physical ego self rather than drawing him closer to the awareness of spiritual Essence.

Furthermore, the now common method of class instruction, in contrast to traditional one-on-one mentoring, is also a new development in the dissemination of yogic teachings, one that holds vastly differing effects. It is impossible to reap the same benefit being one of thirty or a hundred students in a class versus sitting with one's teacher alone in focused study. In the past, great masters taught select students by frequent meditation with them and interpretation of scriptural wisdom, overseeing their daily personal practice. To be effectively understood, Asana needs to be recontextualized in its original role as a supporting part of the full Eight Limbs and taught appropriately to facilitate its intended goal.

The fullness of the meaning of Asana is beyond just creating a strong and supple body. It indicates the ability to sit still, with correct spinal alignment, in seated meditation for extended periods of time. It assumes the ability to quiet the fluctuations of the mind through an inner effort of concentrated calmness. In the tradition of the past, the student would sit for hours at the feet of the master receiving oral teachings and had need of techniques to achieve this stillness and receptivity.

Understood in this way, it makes sense why the original yogis developed thousands of movements that could help them accomplish this goal. Since the spread of the *Hatha Yoga Pradipika*, a yogic text developed approximately 650 years ago, many people equate postures with yoga and have interpreted Asana as any posture that is useful for creating and maintaining a practitioner's well-being or benefitting his flexibility and vitality, in addition to enabling comfortable seated meditation.

If, however, we are to reach the full experience of yoga, which is liberation and unending joy, we must be able to experience the reality of Self through more than just the physical dimension. We need to honor and support our physical bodies but dis-identify with them as the full measure of *who we are*. To do this successfully, a disciplined body and mind are required to enter the state of meditation in which we move beyond association with them into expanded awareness of true Self. This is a complex undertaking, as it is not easy to sit still for any length of time without being distracted by something in the physical realm.

To feel safe and happy, we need both comfort in our physical life and an experiential surety of what lies beyond it. Asana and meditation take us there. A complete explanation of yoga meditation (Dhyana) follows in chapter fifteen.

Energy Channels (Nadis)

The innumerable forms of yoga Asana being offered today all fall under the general term for physical practice that is Hatha Yoga. Asthanga, Kripalu, Iyengar, Anusara, and Vinyasa are just a few forms of Hatha Yoga.

Through some vigorous movement and some gentle stretches, Asana works on the principle of proper energy flow in the body in the same way acupuncture or the martial arts do. This energy runs through thousands of channels (nadis) that distribute it, like blood vessels distribute blood.

By strengthening the nervous system, Asana prepares the body for receiving greater amounts of Life Force Energy. When the nadis are in harmony, the physical body is in balance and we feel fully charged. Every posture we practice can be an experiment in energy movement within the laboratory of our own bodies, where we can observe its subtle effects. Asana teaches us how to seek the point of balance between effort and surrender and between appropriate challenge and self-honoring relaxation.

It teaches us how to create steadiness in the mind, which then influences steadiness in the body.

The physical fitness model of today gauges health through measurements of body fat percentage or performance ability. But the yogic criteria of health are stability and ease in the body assessed by strength, flexibility, range of motion, proper energy flow, ability to withstand change, and skill in focusing and calming the mind. Stability and optimal functioning of the physical body are necessary before we can work effectively with the subtle direction of energy (Pranayama) that is discussed in the next chapter.

Steadiness and Ease

The Sutras on Asana say that the purpose of right posture is to create physical equanimity and comfort. To do this, we practice correct alignment to reset the skeletal system to our best anatomical neutral position in order to optimize the flow of energy throughout the body. We strengthen what we need for foundational support, stabilize what is too open, learn correct breathing patterns and how to control breath, and radiate energy to our extremities to feel a sense of expansion.

These principles affect us not just physically, but mentally as well. When we are energetically or emotionally out of alignment with our center, we cannot think or act clearly. Strength, flexibility, calmness, and ease cultivated through Asana enable us to function better in our jobs, relationships, and creative pursuits. And as we approach the inner practices of concentration

(Dharana) and meditation (Dhayana) we can sit comfortably and quietly with an even mind.

The true yogi is like steel, bendable but unbreakable. Through Asana we learn to stay centered in constantly changing circumstances. This translates into life as we discern the times and ways we need to let go and flow with what is happening, and the times we need to stand our ground and exhibit strength.

A regular practice of Asana helps us build present moment awareness. We apply the principle of right effort (Tapas) to each movement, assessing whether more will force or more surrender is needed, more firmness or more ease. The stability we create physically, mentally, and emotionally through Asana practice renders the ability to have the same presence and fortitude in challenging life situations.

When we are physically aligned with the right laws of nature, balanced in nutrition, exercise, and sleep, dis-ease is less likely to occur. Personal obstacles like agitation, anxiety, apathy, and lethargy fall away. As the body yields unnecessary exertion and tension, we experience joy and comfort in our own skin. We feel free and expansive, able to express the soul within.

Body Awareness for Inner Transformation

In addition to the inner reflections and observances we have already studied through the Yamas and Niyamas, Asana is another tool that can be used for self-transformation and Self-awareness. Because we express our thoughts and feelings through our physical bodies, the way in which we experience various postures provides wonderful material for introspection. Our actions mirror outwardly the beliefs and choices we have already made within.

In general, there are two ways to approach Asana practice: repetition and holding. Postural repetition increases circulation and elimination, overcomes heaviness in the body and mind, and creates adaptability to change. Postural holding promotes inner purification, calms the mind, and encourages stillness. Both are valuable aspects to develop and lead us to greater degrees of happiness and ease in life.

Rather than trying to force a perfect posture, it is important to pay attention to what is happening as we approach it and what arises in the mind as a result. Observe how the mind relates to the body within the pose and after it has been completed. Is there any stress or pain? This is a sure sign of misalignment on some level or over-exertion based in ego. Create appropriate goals. Adapt the practice to your current needs and abilities. Remember, Asana is not meant to foster a greater identification with the body either through pride or frustration. It is meant to create comfort so that we can transcend this basic level of self-knowing.

Asana Categories and Their Benefits

There are general categories found in Hatha Yoga Asana practice, all of which have postures that range from gentle to challenging. Experiment with different forms and styles of Asana practice as well as with the repetition and holding of postures. Feel the difference in the challenge and the benefits. Be watchful for over-exertion that drains energy, and be mindful to apply the principles of peacefulness (Ahimsa) and moderation (Brahmacharya) to each movement.

The general categories of Asana are as follows: Back-bending postures open the chest and front of the torso; they energize the body and increase inhalation. Forward-bending postures open the back, enhance elimination and digestion, and calm the nervous system. Asymmetric or lateral bending postures address unevenness in the body and tightness in the back, shoulders, and pelvic girdle. Twists liberate tension in the spine and release vital energy. They assist digestion and metabolism. Inversions strengthen the spine, deepen respiratory rhythms, and reverse the effects of gravity on the body.

In the same way that the ethical principles of the Yamas and Niyamas create foundational structure for our worldly life, each aspect of Asana practice contributes to our daily experience of balanced ease in our body. Creating proper alignment in the skeletal system helps us feel solidly aligned and supported. Building strength in our arms and legs gives us power and grounding and the ability to move confidently through life. Circulating our flow of energy from center enables fluidity and radiance in our creative expressions. Balance postures offer integration. A steady gaze point (drishti) develops focus. Practicing extension from the feet up to the crown of the head creates a stable foundation that moves to effortless expansion. As such, Asana parallels the overall movement of the Eight Limbs of Yoga.

Before choosing what type of physical yoga Asana to practice, we can recognize that the form we are naturally attracted to and how we do our postures is usually similar to how we approach life. For example, if we are a big energy, Type-A personality who loves action and high intensity environments, we might be naturally drawn to a vinyasa or power-style practice and approach it with fire and determination. However, we could create more internal balance by choosing a calmer, slower style like gentle or restorative yoga, bringing more patience and reflectiveness to our practice. Another example is if we tend toward low energy and a slow-moving pace, we can create more charge and motivation by engaging the faster, flowing practices.

Whatever movement we are doing, the essential element of practice is to stay fully present and notice any inner dialogue. Postures are designed to eliminate restrictions in the body and we are invited to enter these patterns of sensation as a meditative exercise. Witness the experience with a spacious, accepting attitude and watch how this allows the body and mind to open and release. If resistance, distraction, or judgment arises, consider adjusting to a more compassionate, softer attitude about the experience. Contemplate what it means to hold two seemingly opposite qualities at the same time, such as firmness and softness, and how this could benefit other situations in life.

Reflection on the Infinite

The final component in Asana practice and one that is often overlooked in modern classes is this Sutra's direction to reflect upon the Infinite *while* practicing postures. Self-reflection and movement is not to be separated. Anything we do, every thought and every action is therapeutic, neutral, or harmful. And since the body is the vehicle for the Self's expression, Asana can either take us closer to the aim of Self-realization or further from it.

There is a transformative difference between a class that encourages us to use postures as a means of reflection upon the Divine Essence within us, and one that simply uses yoga as exercise. In the true yogi, devotion lives at the heart of every thought and action, so postures are simply another means to that end.

It is not always easy to reflect upon the Infinite when we are feeling great restriction in our physical bodies. But we can practice witness consciousness, and become both the one experiencing Asana, and the one observing inner experience through Asana. Through mindfulness we uncover the subtle obstacles to our mental and physical freedom and we have the opportunity to overcome them.

Overexpenditure in the physical realm is detrimental to our easeful evolution. By balancing energy through our physical practice, we assure an equal or greater amount of energy for the inner spiritual practices that lie ahead. When we relax the ego and engage with the energy of the Universe flowing through us, we experience the Infinite within every breath and every movement. Asana becomes an expression of the Infinite in manifestation and a bridge toward yoga's more contemplative practices. In this way it goes beyond the physical high that movement brings to serve its intended purpose as part of the Eight Limbs, as a building block toward perpetual bliss.

DAILY PRACTICE

Integrate an active practice of right posture and movement into your daily life. Treat the body with detached respect, honoring its needs and creating internal and external equanimity.

- Find the style of Hatha Yoga Asana practice that is right for you to create balance within. Are you someone who is always in high gear, attracted to hot yoga and power core classes? Try a yin or restorative class instead. Or are you a laid-back, more lethargic go-with-the-flow type? Try a vigorous vinyasa class to get your battery charged.

- Create appropriate goals. Adapt the practice to you, not you to the practice. Know and accept yourself, your tendencies, your capabilities, and your rhythms.

- Be sure to get a balanced mix of repetition and holding, as well as backward, forward, and lateral bends, twists, and inversions.

- Notice what happens for you while you are in your postures. Watch for any tension or resistance. If tension, apply acceptance. If resisting, apply gentle focus.

- Remember to include reflection on the Infinite within as an essential focus of your posture practice.

Questions for Further Reflection

Take a moment with your journal now to answer the following questions. Or find a quiet pause sometime today to remember the practice of right posture and contemplate these thoughts further.

- When do you have the inclination to avoid, escape, or distract yourself from the experience of the moment? Practice just being present with whatever is, both on and off your yoga mat.

- Create your personal balance between challenge and compassion. Which one do you practice more naturally with yourself? How about with others?

- Find the still point between your inhale and exhale, between rest and motion, effort and ease. This is the application of right effort (Tapas) and contentment (Santosha). How can you apply these to your work, studies, or family life?

- Assess your well-being according to the yogic criteria:

  - Lightness in the body—Do you have flexibility and good range of motion?

  - Ability to withstand change—Can you adapt quickly to changing circumstances?

  - Stability and comfort in the body—Do you feel strong and at ease in your body?

– Focus in the mind—Is your energy flow even
and your mind calm?

AFFIRMATIONS TO POST AND REMEMBER

Affirmations solidify beliefs in our subconscious minds, creating
a foundation from which we can then manifest positive change
in our outer lives. Repeat these often with strong intensity and
full faith.

- As I practice Asana, I increase my confidence,
  strength, and concentration.

- I am awake to the innate intelligence within my body.

- I see the Infinite in every physical movement, in
  every daily activity.

- With balance as my intention, I create health in
  every cell of my physical being.

- Because my physical experience reflects my
  consciousness, I choose the consciousness of
  love today.

Chapter Twelve

....

Energy Management (Pranayama): Control and Expansion of the Life Force

Guiding and controlling the life force energy currents and
the rhythms of breath stabilizes the mind. Movement
of energy is subtly managed through rhythmic breathing;
inward, outward, in balance, and eventually transcended.
Then one remains anchored in the Inner Light.
Sutras ii.49–ii.53

Just as time management is needed for optimal productivity, energy management is necessary for the optimization of happiness. To understand the scope and practice of Pranayama, it is helpful to break down the word for translation in two slightly different ways. Life Force Energy, called *pran* or *prana* in the

Sutras, is the invisible, intelligent current that flows within us and around us at all times. When the word Pranayama is split as prana and yama, *yama* means "to control." But when it is split as pran and ayama, *ayama* means "to expand." So essentially the practice of Pranayama is the science of both controlling and expanding the energy that activates and organizes our physical bodies.

To function at our peak, this Life Force Energy has to be regulated within and outside our bodies. This is accomplished through focused willpower, visualization, and conscious breathing techniques that help us channel energy in different ways. Through the practice of Pranayama we can decrease tension and anxiety, release emotional and mental stress, recharge physically, and relax deeply.

Everything we are exposed to in the environment affects our level of prana and our ability to take it in and use it effectively. We draw prana from sunlight, clean water, living foods, and all-natural surroundings. We can also benefit from being near yoga masters who have a greater level of prana due to their expanded capacity to control Universal energy. And in advanced practice, Pranayama expands us spiritually toward our true essence by enabling us to perceive consciousness without dependency on breathing at all.

Although sometimes interpreted as "breathing exercises," Pranayama is far more than this. To effectively practice Pranayama, it is essential to intentionally absorb and assimilate vital energy in multifaceted ways. It requires the focused willpower that we explored through Tapas in chapter eight, as well as the ability to visualize ourselves as energetic beings beyond the confines of the physical body.

Scientific Progression of the Eight Limbs

Now we begin to see the scientific progression of the Eight Limbs. Through development of the Yamas and Niyamas, we put our inner and outer lives in order. Next we steady and open the body through Asana, making it an efficient channel of Life Force Energy. This prepares the way for the control and expansion of energy within and beyond the body that Pranayama develops. Then, once energy is intentionally regulated, we can embrace the more subtle practices, such as sensory control through Pratyahara and mind management through Dharana. Each limb supports the next.

As with any practice, we begin where we are and work our way to more over time. With regular Asana practice, we learn to relax and expand in many different circumstances. Over time this will enable all tension, restlessness, heaviness, aching, yawning, blinking, and squirming to subside. Ideally we should be able to sit with ease for thirty minutes or more in order to practice Pranayama without complaint from the body. At the beginning, however, even five minutes of Pranayama practice will yield noticeable results.

Using Breath as a Starting Point

As with most of our practices so far, we begin with the most accessible, outward change possible and then work inward to deeper layers. Because the breath is our constant companion, it is a primary vehicle for the distribution and retention of energy. Yet most people, having no training in Pranayama, breathe inefficiently, taking in shallow, erratic breaths that do not serve to maximize the potential energy resources we need to fuel our lives.

At its most basic level, Pranayama teaches us how to breathe deeper and fuller, and with only a certain number of breaths allotted to any human life, it behooves us to utilize them consciously. Deep breathing calms the restless mind, creating a stronger ability to focus. It also clears out emotions that launch us onto a reactive roller coaster. Now is the time to move beyond unconscious, ineffectual breathing, into an active circulation of breath and prana in our physical bodies.

Anytime we change our breathing patterns, we change our physical experience, our mental state, and the amount of power that is available for our daily activities. This is easily noticed in the simple practice of taking ten deep breaths before speaking when we are upset. By slowing down and bringing intentionality to the breath, the mind calms so we can respond consciously rather than react unconsciously. By far the simplest and best anti-stress medicine we have at our disposal at all times, Pranayama is an invaluable tool for nurturing our mental and physical health.

Take a moment and feel your natural breath. Does it seem small or large? Constricted or free? Shallow or full? Notice the length, rhythm, and sensation of the breath and where you feel it in the body. Make note of any holding or pausing between the inhale and the exhale, or between breath cycles.

Now, place your hands on your belly. Take a big breath in. Was it difficult to get a full breath in? Did the breath get stuck or stop anywhere between the belly and the chest? Did your belly suck inward or did it inflate to allow for the filling up with oxygen? If it sucked inward, you are breathing backwards. The belly should open, like a balloon being inflated when inhaling. Remember, Pranayama is about controlling and *expanding*. Breathing correctly creates space to take in more Life Force Energy.

Now, keep your hands on the belly and notice your exhale. As you let the breath go, does the belly puff out or do the abdominal muscles engage to expel all the air? Was it challenging to fully release the breath or did it explode out in a tremendous sigh?

Ideally the breath should flow evenly and without strain into the inflating belly on the inhalation and out of the relaxing belly on the exhalation. By controlling prana in this way, we also control our experience, mentally, emotionally, and physically. Further breathing techniques are included at the end of the chapter, which enable access to the energy we need in various life situations.

Benefits of Deep Conscious Breathing

Awareness of how we move prana through the breath is a foundational building block of Pranayama. If we did nothing more than learn to breathe slower, deeper, and more evenly, we would increase our health and life span significantly. The strong correlation between the physiology of breathing and length of life is noticeable in the difference in life span between mammals that breathe slowly, like tortoises and elephants, versus those that breathe rapidly like rabbits and mice.

The average human breathes approximately sixteen times per minute, but an advanced practitioner of Pranayama can regulate the movement of energy through breath to less than one cycle per minute. Slowing the breath dramatically like this prolongs life by decreasing stress on the organs and cortisol levels.

In addition to increasing the length of life, Pranayama also promotes a better quality of life experience. On a purely physical level, deep breathing maintains elasticity in lung tissues for greater pulmonary functioning and efficient blood oxygen levels. It also slows the heart rate so blood pressure decreases. It aids digestion through the circulation of fluids to all the organs in the abdomen. It helps eliminate waste by circulating blood to the liver and kidneys, and it aids immune functioning by optimally circulating lymphatic fluid. Consistent deep breathing disposes of carbon dioxide and any buildup of toxins in the bloodstream more efficiently.

With any change in our physical and emotional states, our breathing patterns change naturally. Think of how the breath quickens when we are upset or afraid. By reversing this equation, we see how employing strategic Pranayama practices to effect desired physiological changes gives us a new measure of self-control. Just by changing our breath pattern, we can shift our feeling state. If we are lethargic but need to accomplish a work or school project, we can employ Pranayama that quickens the heart rate and stimulates the brain. If we are feeling anxious and jittery, we can employ a practice that slows the metabolism and racing mind.

Practicing conscious control of the breath lets us bring awareness to patterns of restriction in the body in order to release them. There are hundreds of practices of Pranayama that effect different states of being. Like having a variety of tools in a toolbox, it is helpful to know a variety of practices, so that as we notice what needs attention, we can employ the appropriate Pranayama to overcome blockage and create flow.

Energize, Relax, or Neutralize

On the mental and emotional levels, managing prana through deep breathing helps us relax and lowers the levels of stress hormones. Steady breathing balances the flow of blood to both hemispheres of the brain for positive correlation between the sympathetic and parasympathetic nervous systems, which regulate the spectrum between stimulated brain activity and rest. We feel more control over body and mind, able to integrate emotional responses as they arise.

Studies done at the Harvard Medical School by Herbert Benson, M.D., have shown how stimulating certain areas of the hypothalamus can cause stress, and by activating other areas of the brain, stress is reduced. A steady, slow breath creates what

Benson called an immediate "relaxation response."[11] In contrast, forceful, deep breathing energizes us without the use of artificial stimulants.

Focusing on the breath illuminates our inner landscape. By examining the quality of our exhalation, we see how well we are able to relax and how much we are giving out to the world. Assessing the nature of our inhalation, we determine our level of engagement with life and what we are taking in. We see what needs to change and what we need to let go. If we have been suppressing emotions, conscious breathing will act like a surgeon's knife, excavating that which is creating dis-ease through unhealthy repression or negative beliefs.

Pranayama creates space for inquiry and personal discernment. And it enables us to consciously reprogram for more joy. It gives us the ability to put ourselves into action or rest at will by controlling the involuntary nerves of heart, lungs, and other organs. As we allow vital organs to rest and become replenished with new Life Force Energy, and use our will force to visualize where and how prana is directed, we create the physical and emotional stillness and discipline needed for meditation.

The breath is the link between body, mind, and spirit and as such is the great liberating force, enhancing vitality and creating within us a fuller opening to the endless prana that is available from Source.

11　"Relaxation Response," Mind Body Medical Institute, http://www.relaxationresponse.org/. Accessed January 5, 2015.

Movement of Prana

According to yogic philosophy, Universal Life Force Energy moves through our bodies in the nerve channels (nadis). The word *nadi* comes from the Sanskrit root meaning "to flow." Similar to our circulatory system, the nadis transport subtle energy throughout every cell of the body and just like a river. If there are obstructions to the flow of prana in our system due to illness, mental disturbance, or emotional repression, then we feel stagnant or blocked. By increasing and distributing prana properly, we experience greater health and well-being and prepare for the expansion of our awareness beyond the limited physical body.

The ancient Hindu treatises classify 72,000 nadis and their relationships with the mind. The most important three of these nerve channels are the Ida, the Pingala, and the Sushumna. The Ida is said to transport the masculine energy of the intellect, rational thinking, heat, and the sun. The Pingala channels the feminine energy of feelings and intuition, cooling, and the moon. These correspond to the right and left hemispheres of the brain. The Sushumna is the central channel, running through the body from the root of the spine to the top of the head.

The Ida and the Pingala originate at the base of the spine where a storehouse of latent life force energy (Kundalini) resides. They coil around the central Sushumna like a DNA double helix, similar to the caduceus symbol for the medical profession. Prana moves thru the Ida and Pingala channels in varying degrees depending on both inner and outer conditions and how much self-control (Brahmacharya) we are practicing. If there is too much or too little of either masculine or feminine energy, the physical body will be unbalanced. When these energy channels are in harmony, we feel happier. Through appropriate Pranayama exercises, we create free-flowing channels, and we feel more energetic and optimistic with harmony in our breath and in our lives.

Chakras as Energy Vortexes

The Ida and the Pingala cross each other at seven major energy centers called chakras. Yogic texts describe the chakras like wheels whose spokes radiate the energy and consciousness that have descended into the body out through the spine into all parts of the body, creating the sense-conscious state.

Instructions in the Sutras discuss enhancing prana by regulating inhalation and exhalation, and by suspending the breath with lungs full and lungs empty for greater energy efficiency. As we learn to breathe with stronger intention and control, we prepare ourselves to move beyond the physical experience of being in human bodies, to the experience of being the consciousness within the body. Then in more advanced practices, we learn to increase and directionalize the flow of prana upward through the chakras to the cerebral chakra, or brain, where Divine perception is reawakened. Here we joyfully recognize that we have dominion over the body and are not limited by it in our Soul nature.

To drive the energy to the higher centers of consciousness and maintain it there, we employ locks (bandhas). Like safeguarding our homes by locking the doors when we go out, in Pranayama practice we protect the concentrated movement of prana through bandhas. These are expressed both physically through muscle contraction and energetically through the subtle movement of prana.

The first of the three main energy locks or bandhas is the root lock (Mula Bandha), engaged by contracting the muscles of the pelvic floor and drawing upward internally toward the navel. The second is the abdominal lock (Uddiyana Bandha), which is engaged by drawing the abdominal muscles in and up, hollowing out underneath the lower ribs to seal the prana into the heart center. And third is the throat lock (Jalandhara Bandha), engaged by pulling the chin back and in toward the throat and cervical vertebra. These powerful energy seals should be learned from an experienced teacher.

There are many levels to Pranayama practice, but even the simplest forms consistently used over time allow us to engage with life from awareness based in intentionality and self-control rather than reactivity, self-interest, and survival mentality. Qualities like compassion, generosity, and even love become more accessible as we manage prana correctly. We feel harmonious and happy, because as Patanjali states in the Sutras, the veils over our inner light are swept away and we perceive the Self clearly.

Advanced Stages of Pranayama

Initially the Sutras direct us to modulate the length and depth of breath as well as to focus the mind strongly on the movement of the breath. In more advanced Pranayama practices where the breath is held in differing patterns, novices often strain and then feel a sense of restriction or even panic. Of course this runs counter to the essence of the practice that is meant to calm and clear mental perception, not disturb it. We are advised to engage Pranayama without agitation or tension of any kind. We can only do what we can do today. Like a challenging posture that we accomplish incrementally with regular practice over time, advanced Pranayama reveals itself effortlessly as we perfect our understanding of the mechanics and control of the breath with daily effort.

The *Upanishads* refer to the storehouse of prana held at the base of the Sushumna channel as the Kundalini. This surplus prana is present in all of us and is hundreds of times greater than the energy we normally use. It is depicted as a coiled snake, lying in wait for the time in which we are ready to release our consciousness from the physical domain and reunite it with the spiritual.

Until we can completely control the prana we need and use on a daily basis, we should not try to ignite the release of this surplus, as it can be imbalancing for our daily functioning. Advanced Pranayama should be learned from an experienced teacher who can guide safe and adequate preparation of the body, physically and energetically, for more intensive practices. The gateway for the release of this extra prana opens naturally when the time is right, after much dedicated practice, and should not be forced.

Beyond Breathing

Every human life begins with an inhalation and ends with an exhalation. The final stages of Pranayama come when all effort in the management of the life force through the breath is surrendered. As we contemplate the Infinite as both the breath moving through the body and the awareness of the body being breathed, we recognize that we are not the temporal physical shell but the Spirit within it. And the Consciousness behind the mechanics of breath is the essence of Truth.

When the time is right for our evolutionary advancement, the directional flow of the pranic current reverses from downward to upward in the spine, moving from the physical to the spiritual. Like a mini death, a spontaneous suspension of breath occurs when all prana is drawn inward and upward, aligning us with Higher Consciousness.

Everything stills in body and mind. Perception becomes perfectly clear and the light within shines effervescently. This powerful reversal destroys the barrier of mental ignorance that blocks our awareness, unifying us with pure Consciousness through an uninhibited state of meditation.

This state in which the Life Force Energy disassociates from the breath altogether and prana is felt on a more subtle spiritual level without connection to the physical body is experienced momentarily by many meditators and for indefinite periods of time by masters. The unintentional suspension of breath is the least defined state of Pranayama in the Yoga Sutras and not one to be sought after. We can trust that dedicated practice rather than explanation will take us to this expansive state. We can rest in our consistent, disciplined Pranayama practice, and the deep peace and calm it brings, connecting us effortlessly to Self beyond the physical body.

Daily Practice

Integrate an active practice of energy management into your daily life. These general guidelines should be followed for all efforts in Pranayama. Specific practices are described below.

- Practice in a quiet, well-ventilated space.

- Wear loose clothing, especially around the abdomen, for free functioning of the diaphragm and belly.

- Be sure the stomach is relatively empty so the abdominal muscles are not distracted by digestion.

- Choose any comfortable sitting position on the floor or in a chair where the spine can be straight and the body can be at ease.

- Support the back if needed with a cushion or wall. Support the hips if needed with a pillow or folded blanket. Support the knees if needed with blocks or rolled towels.

- Lengthen the torso and neck to create spaciousness throughout body. Keep the chin parallel to floor. Open the chest by squeezing the shoulder blades together and lifting the sternum.

- Practice for a minimum of five minutes and work up to thirty minutes if desired. Concentration and duration of practice are what determine results.

- Relax. Never strain. Capacity develops naturally with easeful, regular practice.

Visualization to Direct Energy

Visualization and willpower help direct energy during Pranayama. Close your eyes and feel where energy may be low in the body. Visualize the breath moving into that particular body part or circulating throughout the body evenly for healing and balancing. Utilize this in the breathing techniques listed below for maximum result. And employ focus and will to all Pranayama.

Visualization for Higher Consciousness

Visualize the breath moving from the base of the spine up to the crown of the head with each inhalation. See it returning from the crown to the base of the spine on the exhalation. When this imagery is strong, pause at the top of the inhale, visualizing an expansion at the crown of the head, connecting your awareness with Universal Consciousness. Allow any resistance, fear, or doubt to drain into the earth beneath you as you exhale.

Three-Part Breath (Dirga Pranayama)

This basic Pranayama helps to center and ground us. It is also very relaxing. Sit upright and put one hand just below your navel and one hand on your chest. Think of a vase that you fill with water from the bottom of the vase to the middle, then to the top. It is the same with a basic three-part breath. Begin by filling the belly with air first, then the diaphragm, then the chest. When emptying a vase the top empties first, then the middle, then the bottom. So with the exhalation, the chest should empty first, then the diaphragm, then the belly. Abdominal muscles engage to expel all the air out of the body. Visualize tension and stress leaving with each exhalation.

Three-Part Breath Variation (Circumferential Breath)

This Pranayama creates space in the body and expands lung capacity, mirroring how, as we take in more prana, we also expand in our lives. Continue the visualization of the pitcher being filled from bottom to top and emptied from top to bottom. Now add breathing to the outer circumference of the body by placing your hands on the bones at the top of the hips. Start the inhale into the belly and see if you can make the hands on either side of the body move outward with the expansion of air. Move the hands up to the side of the rib cage and expand again. Then place the fingers at your collarbones and make those bones rise with each inhale.

Double Exhale Breath (Sattvic Breath)

A great way to relax and unwind if tension is present is by lengthening the exhale, which triggers a relaxation response by signaling the parasympathetic nervous system. Maintaining awareness of the three-part and circumferential breathing already established, begin to count slowly as you inhale. Do not strain for an unnaturally large inhale. There is no magic number to attain. Just count as you inhale normally. Then as you exhale, pace the out breath so it is twice as long as the inhalation. For example, if your inhale is four counts, try to make your exhale eight counts. If your inhale is twenty counts, make your exhale forty. But do not hold the breath to reach a particular number. The exhalation does not have to be exactly double. Just send the breath out more slowly than it entered.

Double Exhale Breath Variation (Bhramari Pranayama)

To feel the sound vibration of this Pranayama, it is customary to close the eyes and cover the ears with the index and middle fingers. Without counting this time, inhale slowly and naturally through the nose. Then on the longer exhale, with lips closed, make the sound of a buzzing bee, essentially humming the sound of the letter "M." Make the sound as consistent and as long as possible without strain. Repeat for a minimum of ten rounds of breath. Notice how the mind is soothed.

Skull Shining Breath (Kapalabhati Pranayama)

This Pranayama heightens willpower, strength, and intention. It is a heating, activating breath, good for those who are feeling lethargic or down. Maintain a dynamic Pranayama posture with spine erect and torso open. Inhale fully through the nose. On the exhalation, snap the diaphragm back toward the spine, engaging the upper abdominal muscles to expel all the breath rapidly and forcefully through the nose. As the rhythm of the exercise becomes familiar, engage the lower abdominals as well as the diaphragm when you exhale. When this is familiar, finally add the engagement of the muscles of the pelvic floor into a strong root lock (Mula Bandha). Feel strength building in your core and focus building in your mind.

Straw Breath (Kaki Pranayama)

This Pranayama is cooling and reduces tension in the body. It also helps with insomnia as it clears the busy mind. Sit tall with chest and belly open, bring the mouth into the shape of drinking through a straw. Inhale through the mouth and feel the cool air pass across the tongue. Inhale for as long as you can without straining. Then close the lips and exhale slowly through the nose, feeling any bodily tension melting away.

Alternate Nostril Breath (Nadi Shodhana Pranayama)

To balance the overall system, this Pranayama establishes evenness in the nostrils that correspond to the Ida and Pingala nadis. Both energy and calmness are cultivated. Make a fist with one hand. Release the thumb and ring finger. Place the thumb on one side of the nose and the ring finger on the other. Close the right nostril and inhale through the left. Then close the left and exhale through the right. Inhale through the right and exhale through the left. Continue closing off one nostril at a time, always making the change on the exhalation. Do not be concerned if you notice a slight difference in the nostrils at the beginning, one naturally being more open than the other. This can be particularly noticeable if cold symptoms or any nasal obstructions are present. Just do the best you can.

Add a Mantra

Mantras are sounds that tune our minds to a desired outcome. Used consistently, they can completely rearrange mental habit patterns. Once you become familiar with at least one of the above Pranayama exercises, try adding a mantra. Whether you choose a classical Sanskrit mantra like So Hum or Aum, or whether you repeat a quality you wish to cultivate in your native language is up to you.

As you inhale, repeat the mantra silently to yourself. Repeat it again as you exhale. With each breath, become more and more relaxed, finding your way to the still center of your being, to the place of wholeness, integrity, and possibility. Breathe the essence of the mantra or quality you have chosen into your whole body and heart. Notice how it feels to be centered, grounded, present, and aligned. Hold this feeling and enjoy it for a full five minutes.

Questions for Further Reflection

Take a moment with your journal now to answer the following questions. Or find a quiet pause sometime today to remember the practice of energy management and contemplate these thoughts further.

- How do you naturally breathe? Shallow or deep? Longer in or longer out? With difficulty or ease? If your breath is shallow, you may need more self care to replenish energy and revitalize. If you are exhaling too much, you may be giving away too much and need to reevaluate your activities and relationships, practicing Brahmacharya. How does your breath reflect your life at this time?

- Are you aware of times your breath changes or is held back? Which of the Pranayama above would help you feel more at ease?

- How do you feel before, during, and after Pranayama practice? What does this tell you about yourself?

- Shifting your emotional state of being at will creates self-control, intentionality, and equanimity. Which of the above practices could you employ next time you feel angry? Fearful? Sad?

- How else can you manage Life Force Energy through the use of your will?

Affirmations to Post and Remember

Affirmations solidify beliefs in our subconscious minds, creating a foundation from which we can then manifest positive change in our outer lives. Repeat these often with strong intensity and full faith.

- Prana is infinite and I draw from that infinite well.

- I control the use of my energy wisely, with discretion and compassion.

- I breathe consciously to call in all the energy resources I need.

- I expand through my breath, infusing every cell of my body with Life Force Energy.

Chapter Thirteen

....

Inward Turning (Pratyahara): The Peace That Waits Within

*Withdrawal of the senses from
external objects quiets the mind and
enables mastery over sensory experiences.*
Sutras ii.54–ii.55

Throughout most days, we fix our attention outwardly, on our work, families, activities, and natural environments. Our five physical senses (sight, hearing, smell, taste, and touch) are the windows through which outside stimuli enter the mind. We react to these forces, interpret them, and store our perceptions for later. From the moment we wake in the morning until the time we sleep at night, we receive endless information and input from our senses, some of which is pleasant, some not. Whatever stimuli we take in cause emotional and mental responses. These assure our survival, but also support a constant stream of desire and reactivity. And like movement on water prevents us from seeing the depths, these changes keep us from seeing into the depth of our own being. The fluctuation of the senses tosses us around on waves of change between happiness and suffering.

Pratyahara tis the practice of withdrawing temporarily from sensory engagement with the external world in order to calm the restlessness it causes in mind and body. By stilling the continual commentary of the senses, we prepare the way for deeper focus, access our higher wisdom, and enter the expanded awareness of meditation.

As we move further into the Sutras that outline the inner practices of yoga, we must start making choices about the sensory stimulation we surround ourselves with on a daily basis. We will benefit from limiting the intake overload and becoming more selective about what we listen to, read, and watch. This is because the images we receive visually continue to play in our minds, and the words of conversations or songs get stuck in our inner hearing. If these are aggressive or negative, they contribute to our unrest and unhappiness and make the process of turning inward more difficult.

Consider for a moment the sensory stimuli that draw your attention most. Entertainment? News? Food? Sex? Acquisition? If we practice a moment of reflection (Swadhaya), we will notice what leads us toward inner peace and joy and what is simply a passing pursuit of distraction. Interiorization (Pratyahara) begins as we elect moments of silence rather than idle conversation, periods of stillness rather than pointless busyness, and gestures of offering rather than ceaseless craving.

What Mastery of the Senses Entails

A few of the Yamas and Niyamas that we have explored specifically prepare the way for Pratyahara. Yama number one, peacefulness (Ahimsa) is a soul quality that leads us from restless outer blame to harmonious inner responsibility. As we consistently choose a peaceful approach within our own thoughts and in our treatment of others, we find our mind getting quieter and less judgmental. But if we involve ourselves constantly with the world's drama, our internal focus on peace is compromised.

Niyama number one, purity (Saucha) guides us toward the choice of uncomplicatedness and joy. But if we relentlessly pursue fleeting pleasures, we lose control over the senses and they wage a battle within us for satisfaction.

Whenever the mind is identified with the senses, restlessness is the inevitable result. We take charge of our roaming thoughts by conquering the sensory impulses that trigger ideas, obsessions, and habitual actions. Being able to shift focus at will from the sensory and ego-based consciousness to the soul-centered, expanded consciousness develops self-mastery. Sensory withdrawal is a practice of energy control like Pranayama and Brahmacharya.

Noticing desire as it arises and choosing not to give in to it is a way to practice disconnecting from sensory impulses. We do not need to have everything we want. Desire creates perpetual longing for sensory experience and the regeneration of more Karma.

Rather than following desire from one sensory pleasure to the next, we can use desire as a doorway to self-inquiry. Why did that desire arise? When and how often does it arise? By asking ourselves these questions as we watch the sensory draw to indulge in whatever momentary gratification is pulling us, we can assess what sparks craving and address the underlying cause. Learning to be a witness to our internal life is the first step to being able to consciously change it in the direction of happiness.

Bare Attention, Nothing Added

By limiting the senses and being reflective as impulses arise, we recognize unhealthy, repetitive thinking and reactive, volatile emotions that do not serve our highest good. We develop the ability to mindfully watch our own experience and thought with clarity, perspective, and calmness, rather than being so engrossed with it that we are out of control.

With dedicated practice, we liberate ourselves from the unconscious distractions of the senses and use them instead as instruments of the higher mind. Then we are able to engage with sensory pleasures in a grateful yet detached way that neither binds us through addiction or plays us through habit.

By disconnecting from the constant pull of the senses, we develop subtle perception that utilizes the sixth sense of intuition, being able to see or feel things before they have occurred or as they are occurring elsewhere. This inner guidance system helps us with decisions, without lengthy external study or information gathering.

Periodically, throughout the day, notice how many of the senses are engaged. Is there one that could be turned off temporarily? By gaining mastery over the senses, we form the ability to direct them consciously with our mind. We choose when and how to expend our energy.

Unplugged from the ever-changing, overstimulated, external world, our nerves quiet and thoughts recede. Even when we only quiet the senses temporarily, we experience a vision of existence much greater than the grasping senses show us. With our focus directed inward, we simply hold gratitude for the origin of all sensory pleasure, which is Divine Source. Through Pratyahara we move closer to soul consciousness.

The happiness that comes from this form of self-mastery is far greater than the fleeting enjoyment of the senses. We experience a clear inner palette through which to relate to the world and other people. Mastery of the senses is the basis of true mental health and inner equilibrium.

Focus on the Third Eye

In daily life, the majority of information we gather from the outside is done through the sense of sight. By closing our eyes and changing our visual focus to a point within, we immediately begin the journey toward interiorization of consciousness. To do this, the point of focus (drishti) recommended by yogis is the metaphoric third eye, the center of concentration, will, and creative thought, found more or less near the point between the eyebrows.

As discussed previously, the two main nerve channels, the Ida and the Pingala, transport energy throughout the body. Initiating at the base of the spine, they cross each other at the seven major chakra points as they wind up the Sushumna or central axis. They finally join at the sixth chakra or third eye.

The practice of intently gazing internally to this point, so that the closed eyelids become motionless, is called the Sambhabi Mudra. A mudra is a gesture that affects a particular quality, like creativity, by stimulating certain nerves, in this case those associated with the pineal gland, also known as the pineal eye. French philosopher René Descartes, considered the "father of modern philosophy," described the pineal gland as the principal seat of the soul and considered it equivalent to the yogic third eye.

The pineal gland is a small endocrine gland responsible for our sleep patterns and circadian rhythms. It rests directly between the two hemispheres of the brain in diagonal alignment between the third eye and the medulla oblongata, the posterior part of the brain that tapers off into the spinal cord. Yogis believe the medulla oblongata to be the spot where Life Force Energy enters the human body. Connecting our awareness between the medulla and the third eye creates a powerful pull of energy toward higher consciousness.

The Sambhabi Mudra is accomplished by gently turning the closed eyes upward, focusing at a point between and just slightly above the eyebrows. There is no need to cross or strain the eyes in any way. Concentrating within, then we utilize Pranayama to draw greater energy through the medulla and link it to the third eye, center of intuitive soul wisdom. In this way, we join our physical and spiritual worlds. By temporarily closing down the windows to the outside world, and turning our focus inward, we find the simplicity and joy of stillness within. Then we can bring this back to our outer lives.

What Waits Within

It is important now to create a quiet space and time in our home for dedicated practice of Pratyahara and the other limbs that are to follow. Interiorization takes concerted effort and if ambient noise from traffic, neighbors, or family members is distracting, it can be helpful to wear earplugs. As the energy currents that flow outward from the ears are trained to focus inward, delicate inner sounds will be perceptible. Sometimes the prana moving through the nerve channels can be heard as subtle Divine music similar to the sounds of harps, bells, or waves. And when our own mental voice gets quiet, the still, small voice of wisdom speaks intuitionally to us. In deep stillness, eventually the great vibration of creation, the Cosmic Aum, is audible.

For some visual people colors and lights will display on the field of inner vision when concentration is deep. And for the more kinesthetic, currents of energy may be felt in the spine and brain. The Sutras caution us not to seek phenomena but to enjoy it without attachment if it arises spontaneously.

The most important thing to focus on as we withdraw attention from our senses and concentrate within is simply our personal experience of Spirit as our true nature. The system of the

Eight Limbs leads us into this reunion of sense to soul, or individual consciousness to Universal Consciousness.

Effects of Pratyahara

If we remain identified solely with the body and its sensory pleasures, our ego will run our lives and we will struggle and suffer as a result. Through practice of Pratyahara, we gain control over our senses, moods, and thoughts. We regain the inner perception of our Divinity, which allows us to function with more joy in our humanity, as we remain focused on the bigger picture of life. We have less reactive and happier relationships, more non-attached fun and contentment in our activities, and more clarity and ease in our work. Established in soul-centered awareness, perceiving Spirit within and without, we engage empathetically with others and seek the common good rather than just serving our own impulses and desires.

When spiritual perception becomes our primary goal, then any challenge life throws at us will not embitter us, make us despair, or entice us to retaliate. It will simply push us more intently toward higher consciousness. As we maintain internal focus, we will find freedom in our bodies as they become unfettered by sensory habits. In addition, we will enjoy a blissfulness that is beyond all physical experience.

The Sutras assure us that through the combination of Pranayama and Pratyahara, the inner light of Truth is revealed. We achieve peace and contentment and are able to bring this unshakeable serenity back into daily life as a lightness in our overall being.

DAILY PRACTICE

Integrate an active practice of interiorization into your daily life. Recognize that as much or more of life lies within as it does without, and find a balance of functional living combined with peaceful withdrawal.

- Take mini breaks during your day to change the channel of your attention from outside to inside. Simply stop what you are doing, close your eyes, and notice what sensations or emotions are coursing through your body.

- Become a witness to contents of your mind. Practice watching a thought float in the mind without allowing it to flow onto the next thought.

- Create a space in which you can have silence. Close down all the senses and approach being still.

- When practicing Asana, try doing your postures with your eyes closed. Notice the experience of moving from the inside out instead of from the outside in.

- Practice Sambhabi Mudra. With eyes closed, focus your inner gaze at the third eye point. Hold your attention there as long as you can. Then with open eyes, focus there again, holding steady attention as long as possible. The practice of directing our attention to the third eye in any gap of time that we do not have to be focused outwardly helps build the discipline of Pratyahara.

Questions for Further Reflection

Take a moment with your journal now to answer the following questions. Or find a quiet pause sometime today to remember the practice of sensory withdrawal and contemplate these thoughts further.

- Which sense pulls on you the most? What could you accomplish if this sense was being directed by a clear mind, rather than constantly creating agitation in your thoughts or body?

- In what way do your senses create difficulty in relationships? How can this form of self-mastery improve your relationships?

- Which Yamas and Niyamas do you need to practice more in order to support the effort of Pratyahara?

- When you close your eyes and draw attention inward, what do you see on the inner screen? What do you hear with the inner ear?

Affirmations to Post and Remember

Affirmations solidify beliefs in our subconscious minds, creating a foundation from which we can then manifest positive change in our outer lives. Repeat these often with strong intensity and full faith.

- I move effortlessly inward to a state of stillness and observation.

- My senses respond to the wise direction of my highest Self, not the fleeting desires of my ego.

- By controlling my sensory impulses, I create space to experience beauty and fulfillment within.

- I know my Self more fully as I quiet the external impulses and listen to my soul within.

Chapter Fourteen

....

Focused Attention (Dharana): Developing Concentration

Focusing the mind on one point of
attention within is concentration.
Sutra iii.1

Multitasking is accepted as a necessary part of modern daily life. Although at times it fulfills the intended benefit of efficiency, it often comes at the price of lower-quality results and higher stress levels. If we allow ourselves to be in more than one place at a time, doing one thing but thinking about another, spending time with a person but daydreaming about someone else, we will never give our best. Far greater depth, success, and fulfillment come when we focus our full attention on the people and projects we are attending to. Also, by retraining ourselves to be mindful of what is happening right now, rather than occupied mentally with thoughts of the past or the future, we experience this moment more richly and completely.

This Sutra explains that single-pointed devotional attention brings our restless, wandering thoughts under control, allowing us to feel more serene, clear-minded, and creative. The practice of building steadfast focus on one thing that inspires love and devotion is called Dharana. It paves the way to enter the deep stillness of meditation and lasting happiness.

Single-Pointed Attention

Lack of proper concentration is the root cause of many failures in life. As explored in the last chapter on Pratyahara, sensory stimuli, as well as the feelings and thoughts associated with those stimuli, distract us in multiple directions all day long. Development of the ability to unplug the senses prepares the way for devotional concentration. Only when the senses have been brought under control of the higher mind can we sit still without being pulled around by sensations, desires, and habits.

To concentrate means to gather attention at one point. If we concentrate exclusively on one thing at a time, we increase both our creative efficiency and our loving presence. Our families, our spiritual studies, and even our alignment in Asana class will all benefit from undivided attention.

On a daily basis, the mind is in continuous movement, creating plans, analyzing conversations, checking to-do lists, reacting to external stimuli. The mind runs through information, personal experience, memories, inference, and intuitive insights constantly. It is ever-dividing concepts and experiences into positives and negatives, things to be desired or things to be avoided. Sri Swami Satchidananda calls the practice of Dharana taming the wild monkey mind. And like taming or training anything, this takes patience, commitment, and repeated effort.

The practice of Dharana is accomplished by binding the mind through concentration to one thought, idea, or concept, specifically one that arouses devotion, awe, or love within us. By using devotion (Iswara Pranidhana) to direct our attention through love, we align with the strongest focusing force. No material pleasure can ever deliver the happiness we receive through devotion.

Directing the mind toward our chosen focal point, regardless of external or internal distractions that may arise, builds mental stability, just as Asana practice builds physical stability. If we learn to concentrate completely, we clear the mind and intuitive perception dawns. We can then move through outer circumstances with discernment, knowing our right decisions and actions. Eventually the mind becomes like a tranquil lake, without the ripples of habitual thought, and we feel pure peace and clarity of understanding.

This devotional focus (Dharana) combined with the previous practice of sensory withdrawal (Pratyahara) primes us for entering the state of stillness that is meditation (Dhyana).

Focus Training Techniques

Think of the development of concentration like a muscle that needs to be strengthened, similar to a physical muscle. If we are just beginning to lift weights, we certainly would not expect to lift 200 pounds on the first try. If we are just learning Asana, we should not expect to accomplish an advanced yoga posture immediately. Only through diligent, daily effort do we find ourselves at our intended destination of strength, balance, or concentration.

To build the muscle of concentration, it is helpful to learn techniques to help us relax physically while remaining alert and peaceful at the same time. Any tension in the body will create disturbance in the mind as well, preventing single-pointed focus. But when the body and mind have an ongoing dialogue, necessary adjustments for comfort can be made quickly when the time comes to practice Dharana with intention.

Start with the common sense basics to put the body in balance. Exercise regularly. Eat a moderate diet of fresh, wholesome foods. Eliminate excess stimulation like background radios or televisions. Get a massage or other bodywork to relieve long-term stress that has built up. Pay attention to the body's needs for rest and sleep. Listen within instead of pushing through physical signals of exhaustion. Balance work and play.

As a specific tension-releasing technique, periodically throughout the day take a deep breath in and squeeze all the muscles of the body. Then exhale and let all the tension and stress go. Repeat as needed.

Once the body is relaxed yet still awake and alert, then it is time to relieve the mind. Train yourself to think just one thought at a time. Do not mentally go around and around about problems. Do not interrupt others when they are speaking in order to get a point across. Choose books that require concentration. Set worries down often. And sometimes, just be quiet, doing nothing at all.

As a specific mind-relieving and focusing technique, try this experiment. Close your eyes and breathe into the quality of peace. Concentrate on the word peace. Feel your entire body relaxing, becoming calm and serene. If you notice stress somewhere in the body, say to yourself, "I am breathing peace in here," and visualize that body part receiving rejuvenation. Then say silently, "I am breathing stress out now" and visualize the body part releasing all tension. "I am breathing in peace. I am breathing out stress. I am breathing in peace. I am breathing out stress. I am breathing. I am peace. I am breathing. I am peace. Peace. Peace." Place wholehearted attention and feeling into the experience of peace filling your being. Allow all else to fall away as just that energy becomes pervasive in your mind.

When we first begin Dharana practice, unrelated and distracting thoughts will come and go through the mind. Use willpower to compassionately retrieve your focused thought. Both firmness and love are needed, as if calling a small, rambunctious child to sit beside you. With time and dedication, we will build the muscle of concentration, reaping benefits of success and ease. Remember muscles are built gradually. Consider all effort to be progress.

Deeper Than Contemplation

In some translations of the Sutras, Dharana is defined as contemplation, yet it is actually beyond contemplative introspection. When we combine concentrated thought with an attitude of devotion (Iswara Pranidhana), our love makes a profound difference. Dharana practice is not intellectual analysis. It is quieting the mind through one-pointed focus until thought drops away completely and we are left naturally in devotional meditative stillness.

In order for this to occur, Dharana practice must be dedicated focus on something uplifting, inspiring, or faith-inducing. Anything that awakens love, awe, or joy will do. Yoga philosophy acknowledges Universal Consciousness as manifest in all things, therefore, according to personal faith, we can choose anything that invokes love in our hearts and devotion in our souls. The focusing image is a way to train the mind into single-pointed attention, like a bridge from outer to inner awareness. Eventually, like all thought, it dissolves as we enter meditation.

Experiment in this way. Call to mind the image of something or someone that you love. Sink into the energetic feeling of loving as you did into the feeling of peace before. When the quality of love becomes your tangible internal experience, hold awareness completely on that and allow the image of the beloved to fade into the background of the mind. Recognize that you are one with this love that flows through you, the pure energy of Source Love.

Other good tools for focusing are mantras or sacred words infused with spiritual meaning, like Aum or So Hum. Images of a preferred deity or Self-realized master, or any spiritual quality like compassion or peace also work. The devotional aspect of yoga is called Bhakti, through which we personally realize the presence of and our unity with the one Beloved.

From Focused Awareness to Full Expansion

By binding thought to one devotional center, we release the mind from its daily work and allow perception to move beyond thought, into pure experience. Energy flows where focus goes. If we pour focus into love, joy, and devotion, then these become our experience. Eventually this focused awareness leads us beyond personal ego-driven experience, through the portal of stillness into the expansive field of pure Consciousness, wherein we become simultaneously aware of everything from the smallest atom to the infinite cosmos. The Sutras indicate that as we release the agenda of individual self into the realm of infinite Self, we experience grace and liberation from all our difficulties. This master level awareness is what the Eight Limbs of Yoga are moving us toward.

From here we delve into the subtler spiritual realms of yoga practice. Any haphazard approach must be replaced with whole-hearted commitment and willingness to stay the course no matter what we see in outer results in a month, a year, or even more. Many people try something a few times and feel no result, so they walk away, determining that it does not work. This is like digging a few shallow wells instead of one deep well. Only patient diggers will find the life-sustaining water. It is useful to commit to one focusing technique for three to six months to give the practice of Dharana a chance to solidify. Nothing is accomplished overnight, much less full liberation! A dedicated habit of focus and concentration in both our daily activities and in our formal yoga practice is required.

It is important to recognize, too, that everyone's movement toward expanded consciousness unfolds at a different pace, according to current effort, Karma, attitude, and openness. As the Serenity Prayer suggests, we accept the things we cannot change, have courage to change the things we can, and employ the wisdom of discernment to know the difference.

Summarizing again the building blocks of the Sutras up until this point, we see that the integrated Yamas and Niyamas give us increasing tranquility internally and in our environments. Asana creates steadiness in our body, and Pranayama controls and expands our energy flow. Pratyahara restrains the senses so we may establish a fertile field on which to cultivate the seeds of devotion. These first five Limbs can and should be practiced simultaneously.

The last three limbs build more concretely in order upon each other. Dharana develops concentrated focus into a devotional awareness in which we feel inner peace and enter meditative stillness (Dhyana). With regular and consistent practice, concentration and stillness create the space for mergence with Universal Consciousness (Samadhi). Then we live, move, and breathe in a state of inner tranquility and joy.

DAILY PRACTICE

Integrate an active practice of focused attention into your daily life. Gather your awareness into the now and experience each moment of life more completely. Offer this devotional concentration to the Divine in all that you do.

- Practice mindfulness by doing just one thing at a time and focusing your entire attention on it.

- Notice when you feel your attention drifting or fragmenting. Attempt to bring it back to single-pointed focus on whatever is happening in the moment. Do this often throughout the day to build awareness and the muscle of concentration.

- Choose carefully something devotional that will assist you in holding this deep inward focus. This could be a mantra, a quality you wish to cultivate, a sacred word, an image of a loved one, or a beloved representation of the Divine—whatever brings you joy. Commit a certain period of time each day to sitting still with this focus.

- The sound of Aum represents the vibratory energy inherent in all creation, and chanting it is a powerful bridge between individual and Universal Consciousness. Try chanting Aum softly, then more loudly until you feel the vibration moving through and aligning your body, mind, and soul.

QUESTIONS FOR FURTHER REFLECTION

Take a moment with your journal now to answer the following questions. Or find a quiet pause sometime today to remember the practice of devotional focus and contemplate these thoughts further.

- In what aspect of your life is it easiest to retain focus and concentration? Family life? Work? Spiritual practice? Athletics? Hobbies? Why do you think this is?

- In what aspect of your life is it most difficult to attain pure concentration? How could you apply what you feel in your focused activities to the ones that feel less so?

- What do you think would change in your primary relationships or projects if you brought more single-pointed attention to them?

- How can focusing on an aspect of the Divine bring you into deeper relationship with true Self?

AFFIRMATIONS TO POST AND REMEMBER

Affirmations solidify beliefs in our subconscious minds, creating a foundation from which we can then manifest positive change in our outer lives. Repeat these often with strong intensity and full faith.

- I experience deep peace within as I cultivate focused awareness.

- Single-pointed attention helps me be more creative, loving, and present in my life.

- I connect to Source through devoted focus, an open heart, and a quiet mind.

- As I focus on love, my busy mind rests.

Chapter Fifteen

··························

Meditation
(Dhyana): The State
of True Stillness

A sustained concentration on the Divine
Light within is meditation.
Sutra iii.2

There is no shortage of proof these days of the benefits of all forms of meditation. Studies have documented decreased stress, fear, tension, and worry; increased concentration and learning capacity; lowered blood pressure and better immune functioning; improved relaxation and pain management; better overall health and increased youthfulness; stronger performance at work and in sports; and a greater sense of altruism, peacefulness, and lasting joy. These results are consistent regardless of the type of meditation one practices, whether based on mindfulness, loving kindness, guided visualization, transcendence, or devotional concentration, such as yoga meditation.

It is important to recognize, however, that none of the above is given as the goal or intent of yoga meditation (Dhyana) as written about in the Sutras. Although innumerable physical benefits come from the practice, yoga meditation is solely intended as the pathway to egoless stillness wherein we reunite our individual consciousness with Divine Conciousness. To be a yogi is to meditate.

Mistakenly, many people think of yoga and meditation as two separate practices. Yet the Sutras clearly describe meditation as the core of the teachings and the culmination of all practices upheld by the previous limbs. By cultivating a balanced lifestyle, proper energy management, sensory control, and focused attention, we prepare ourselves for the state of pure awareness that is meditation (Dhyana). It is here we experience the intended purpose and goal of yoga, the stilling of the fluctuations of the mind and the expansion of consciousness to its natural omniscience and joy.

Purpose of Life

The root of the word yoga is *yug*, meaning "to yoke or unite," indicating the union of personal and Universal Consciousness, or the union of soul and Spirit. The practices of the Eight Limbs of Yoga are a grand experiment with the spiritual laws that take us to this unified state, which we conduct in the laboratory of our lives. Like the yogis and rishis of the past, we discover proof of the theories by the changes that manifest in our own behavior and thought. Through all the practices discussed so far and culminating in meditation, we come to know the Divine within. Direct personal contact trumps any philosophical speculation. According to yoga philosophy, this reunion is the whole purpose of life!

The Eight Limbs of Yoga practiced in our daily lives deliver documentable results of permanent happiness and fulfillment. Through reconnection with our Divine Self, we are freed from all suffering and personal desire. We exist in unending peace and ever-present joy, perfect awareness, pure wisdom, and unconditional love.

Beginning Meditation

In order to enter the state of being that is Dhyana or true meditation, we must be able to transcend physical sensations long enough to liberate our awareness from its usual body identification. Through our earlier practices of Brahmacharya, Asana, and Pratyahara we have begun the process. Now as we approach formal seated meditation, we begin with a posture that allows the optimal flow of energy through the chakras to Higher Consciousness.

The first step in accomplishing this is to make the body as comfortable as possible while maintaining a vertical spinal column. Position of the spine is most essential because compression in the vertebra can prevent the proper movement of energy to the centers of higher perception that awaken during prolonged practice. Think of the spine like a garden hose that, if it gets pinched, will not allow the water to run through.

If no handicaps prevent us from having an erect spine, it is best to maintain this posture throughout yoga meditation. Leg position is not as important, so experimentation is helpful to determine our most comfortable seat. Sitting in a chair with feet placed evenly on the ground is one option. Kneeling over a small bench or cushions works for some. Sitting cross-legged with the hips supported enough to enable the knees to drop forward is the classic yoga meditation posture. Advanced versions of seated meditation posture include full lotus or heels aligned below the navel point. By practicing various Asana to create steadiness and ease in the body, we will find a seat that supports us well, so we can forget the body entirely in meditation.

Meditation Techniques

Next we must determine to shut out the concerns of the world temporarily. Detach sensory awareness from the outer world. Throw everything out of thought except the technique being used to focus the mind, aided by devotional love. At first, it is normal for thoughts to be restless and for the subconscious to throw up distracting and disturbing images. Practice being a witness to intruding thoughts without judging them. Simply recognize patterns of distraction. "Ah, here is a repetitive thought. It is based in fear. Here is old resentment. Here is attachment to outcome." Allow them all to arise and fade away without much attention. Use willpower to stay single-pointed on your mantra or Pranayama, and focus intently on the third eye (Sambhabi Mudra). Be determined to succeed.

The mind is a repository of all past experiences, so like a glass of muddy water it is a murky swirl until we sit in stillness long enough for the dirt to settle and the clarity of consciousness to return. With continued effort to train our thoughts to one point of focus, the tiresome intrusions eventually recede. We move into a place of spaciousness in the mind and ease in the body and breath. By disengaging habitual patterns and responses, we break free from unhealthy ways of thinking and acting. We become lighter, freer, more understanding, and more compassionate with others and ourselves. We watch the train of thoughts go by and see that on the other side of the tracks is joy. It is already there, right now. We just have to clear the way to receive its blessing.

Although the mind has value in the domain of intellectual learning, we must tell it to rest as we enter soul territory within the experience of stillness. Whatever we have been pondering before meditation will still be there for the mind after meditation—in fact, in a clearer, more organized way. In silence we find intuitive clarity, increased creativity, and an overall feeling of happiness that is not attached to any particular circumstance or person.

Eventually, all association with time, space, body, and mind falls away. We overcome attachment to and identification with the sensory self and ego. We suspend the outward flow of energy to the world around us and experience an inward and upward flow through which we know ourselves as individualized reflections of the Divine. Our focused attention melts into a peaceful awareness where no agenda remains beyond being and listening. Meditation becomes a receptive place of rest and renewal. In the stillness within, we carry our portable happiness.

Never Give Up

Although much within us needs to be emptied out to come into the still space of meditation, it is far from a void once we are there. Overflowing with creativity, it is an active, pulsing field of potential being. By uniting our personality-based consciousness with the Infinite Consciousness, we experience this magnitude within.

To reach this state of joyful renewal, perseverance is key. Even if our meditations are only five short minutes out of a 1,440-minute day, absolute dedication is necessary. If meditation remains optional in our mind, it will never become habitual.

Think of it this way. We do not question whether or not to eat or brush our teeth daily. So if we aspire to the freedom and joy that the Eight Limbs of Yoga promise, we cannot question whether or not to meditate. Unwavering commitment is required for spiritual success. We must keep our appointment with the Divine Self to cross the inner bridge to lasting happiness.

Several things help. Create a space that is dedicated to meditation. Even a small corner of a room with a comfortable seat and a personal token of devotion to the Divine is a good start. This space will hold the energy of serenity that is cultivated during practice. Start now! People let years pass, saying, "I will do it tomorrow," but procrastination kills good intentions. Have patience and persistence. Recognize that this is a long-term endeavor, not one of immediate gratification.

Ideally we should meditate twice a day at generally the same time to establish a positive habit. Once a week, a longer meditation is beneficial. If we were studying physics or learning tennis or the violin, we would think nothing of dedicating whole days to the pursuit. Finding a group meditation can also be a tremendous support and boost to individual practice. Even during challenging times that disrupt our routine, we can offer something to our practice. When life is chaotic, this is exactly when we need to cling to our meditation time the most. No matter what circumstance comes along to derail us, a true yogi never gives up.

Meditation is not easy for anyone. Faith in the process and trust that results will come eventually, coupled with the true spirit of devotion, are what make the biggest difference. Spirit watches the heart. If we are putting in the effort through wholehearted devotion while we are practicing, we are progressing whether or not evidence is obvious.

Signs of Progress in Meditation

With consistency and a trusting attitude, we can expect certain signs of progress in meditation. The key is not to look for them or be attached to results coming in any particular order or time frame.

Typical results begin with a feeling of increasing peacefulness. It becomes easier to sit for longer periods of time with unbroken focus and bodily ease. This calmness transcends our time of practice and then begins to infuse daily life. We find ourselves less reactive to outer circumstances, and more joyful for no apparent reason. The ego relaxes and intuitive wisdom arises, providing guidance for our lives. This promotes greater efficiency in daily life, both physically and mentally. We shed bad habits more quickly and nurture spiritual qualities with ease.

For some people, internal lights or sounds occur, as discussed in chapter thirteen. As we strengthen our concentration, eventually thought gets quiet. The channel of our awareness opens to the direct realization of Truth. When this occurs, we are no longer disturbed by worry, anger, fear, or any other imbalanced mental state.

Over time, we find that what used to require discipline is now filled with natural pleasure. We feel connection with and compassion for all mankind. We are receptive and loving when we know the Divine within ourselves and all around us.

The Self Patiently Waits

As we go deeper into the still point of meditation, sometimes fear arises as we notice the disappearance of self, the "I" that we have believed is who we are. The ego self fears that if it is not thinking, acting, choosing, or processing, that "we" will not be. However, if we relax into the detached stillness, we perceive something beyond the petty, fleeting thoughts and feelings that we identify with most of the time. With sustained practice of meditation techniques, fleeting moments of peace become longer and we exist in the space beyond doing, where we know ourselves as more than our thoughts, feelings, and actions.

Here we recognize that we are not separate and alone, but intimately one with all and totally safe. We perceive that which we truly are, the Consciousness that watches and holds all of the experiences and perceptions we know as life. We realize a realm of pure potential and freedom. If we can fully surrender separate self at this point, we enter communion with the Divine Self through loving devotion.

We do not have to believe this to meditate. We meditate in order to prove this through personal experience. When our consciousness merges with the One Consciousness, all we feel is the blissful state of union. Once there, devotion to this essential Self blossoms into unconditional love.

DAILY PRACTICES

Integrate a practice of stillness into your daily life. In mind, body, and soul, become willing to let the world fall away so you can enter the pure awareness within. A meditation practice is built one day at a time.

- Throughout the day, pause and sit in silence for a moment or two. Draw attention inward and recognize the sacredness of each moment.

- Commit to daily meditation. Create a small space that is just for your practice. Determine a regular time that you will not be disturbed. Even the smallest commitment will reap huge rewards.

- Maintain an ordered practice. Like any ritual that cues the subconscious toward a desired outcome, it is helpful to create a structure for meditation time. Here is an example of a sample practice:

  - Prepare the body for easeful sitting through Asana or gentle stretches to relieve tension.

  - Turn off the phone and set a timer for fifteen to thirty minutes.

  - Find a comfortable seat, maintain an erect spine, and relax. Keep the chin parallel to the ground and hands resting gently in the lap.

  - Offer a prayer of intention or chant a devotional song.

  - Practice Pranayama to regulate energy flow through the breath. Choose any from the chapter on Pranayama or try this simple pattern for ten repetitions. Inhale for ten counts, hold the breath for ten counts, and exhale for ten counts.

  - Discipline the inner gaze to Sambhabi Mudra, the third-eye point of concentration.

  - Move into silent repetition of a breath-coordinated mantra such as So Hum, Sat Nam, or Aum, mentally repeating one syllable with each section of breath. Or breathe in and out with a quality such as love or peace.

- Continue for a period of time until you feel
  yourself move into stillness, no thought, pure
  being. Stay in this receptivity and enjoy the
  peacefulness as long as possible. If it ends
  too quickly, return to Dharana, focusing on
  devotion, awe, and love.

- Conclude with a prayer of gratitude or an
  affirmation of your Divinity and wholeness.

QUESTIONS FOR FURTHER REFLECTION

Take a moment with your journal now to answer the following
questions. Or find a quiet pause sometime today to remember the practice of meditation and contemplate these thoughts
further.

- Our experience is determined by the level of
  consciousness we operate from. Which is in
  control for you right now, ego or soul?

- If it is the ego, you may find yourself judging
  or criticizing; worrying or doubting; shaming,
  manipulating, or instilling guilt; comparing yourself
  to others; wavering in decisions or feeling fearful;
  being reactive, impulsive, or defensive. How do you
  suffer as a result of ego consciousness?

- When soul intuition is in charge, you will accept changes with ease and trust life's process; feel centered regardless of chaos in your environment; be unattached to any particular outcome; feel at peace and able to express love even when others disappoint you; know your right direction and answers even without conclusive information and feel a sense of interconnectedness to all life. How can you invite this state of consciousness more often?

- Review all the limbs covered so far. How well are you integrating them in daily life?

AFFIRMATIONS TO POST AND REMEMBER

Affirmations solidify beliefs in our subconscious minds, creating a foundation from which we can then manifest positive change in our outer lives. Repeat these often with strong intensity and full faith.

- I release thought and action to experience a deeper level of being.

- In stillness I know my true Self.

- Peaceful, intuitive awareness is mine as I cultivate stillness within.

- I am pure peace and joy.

Chapter Sixteen

....

Liberation
(Samadhi): Achieving
Lasting Bliss

All sense of separation dissolves when
individual consciousness merges with Universal
Consciousness. This union is liberation.
Sutra iii.3

We have traveled far along the path of *True Yoga* and now are
near the end of our journey. Like those who trek to the summit
of a majestic mountain, through integration of the practices of
the Eight Limbs of Yoga, we receive a higher perspective on life.
Although spiritual progress is subtle and everyone experiences
their evolution in different ways and times, we know we are getting closer to our destination when we feel a daily conviction to
overcome anything that stands in our way of lasting happiness.

Obstacles presented by our karma or the ego no longer discourage us and our efforts remain diligent. We are sure that our progress toward sustainable joy is happening with each hurdle we surmount.

Time to Ignite

Like a stove burner filled with grease and dirt that will not ignite, the light of our soul is blocked by ego-centered living. Bad habits, negative thoughts, identification with the sense of a separate self, all keep us in a less-than-joyful experience. However, the tests of life are never meant to stop us but rather to make us look away from our egoistic belief in self-sufficiency and toward the true Source of all strength and wisdom. We choose which charts the course for our lives, the ego or the Soul.

As long as we are identified with the body, mind, and emotions, we remain in ignorance (Avidya) of our infinite power and beauty. When we are being dictated by the ego, we feel limitation, frustration, and a longing to be free. The self-centered consciousness of "I, me, mine" keeps us from the brilliance of our soul. We suffer while the Divine Self waits patiently for us to clean up the mess we have made and prepare ourselves to be vessels of Divine Light. We are sparks of this Divine Source of Light and it is time to ignite.

Happiness Is a Choice

Intuitively we sense the freedom that awaits us. We innately want to go home to abide in our natural state of love and peace, even more so on days that we feel trapped in challenge and delusion. In fact, it is the very reason we constantly seek happiness.

The moment we see through the illusions of false happiness centered in the desires and attachments of human life, we open to a new reality. A vast world of love and joy exists already within and around us. We do not have to create it. We just have to remove the veil of ignorance that hides it. This requires a dauntless will to place the ego in service to the soul, allowing little self to be absorbed into the Divine Self. There is no loss or lack in this movement, rather an expanding enthusiasm for all that is.

The Sutras indicate that if for just one moment we release all thought and merge into complete awareness of our true nature, we will be overcome with joy. Sustaining this awareness, we could then inhabit our limited human body with an awareness of our infinite nature and not be frustrated by this transitory experience. When consciousness realizes that it is not really trapped by the temporal, then it can relax within the experience and enjoy the hidden joy in everything. To tap into this infinity within is why we study, live ethically, practice Asana, meditate, and seek Self-awareness. The entire teaching of the Eight Limbs of Yoga points to this bliss.

Being versus Doing

The more devotedly we practice the Eight Limbs of Yoga, the quicker we overcome the ego and brighten into the awareness of our true blissful nature. Yet we have come to the end of the limbs that can be "practiced" per se. Instruction in effort ends at the sixth limb of concentration (Dharana). At this point, *being* replaces *doing*. The last of the Eight Limbs of Yoga is not a practice that we manage, but rather the result of continuous practice of all the other limbs and a gift of grace when we are ready to receive it. The Sutras describe how deep concentration naturally merges into meditation, which then spontaneously leads to liberation (Samadhi), the full union with pure Consciousness.

Although attainable, Samadhi is considered indescribable in its fullest measure. Because the identity of small self disappears, there is nothing left to describe and define its experience, no more observer to describe the experience of what is observed. The Sutras say the instrument of seeing (i.e., the body) is no longer confused with the seer (i.e., the Self).

Masters who have entered the boundless expansion of Samadhi have given us some partial descriptions of this state of being so that we can have a reference point. In Samadhi, they say, there is no more need for effort, no more resistance, no more sorrow, no more attachment, and no more pain. Unending joy, pure peace, a selfless desire to serve others, intuitive wisdom, unconditional love, and compassion, and a constant flow of energy are ever-present. In this state of awareness, joy flows from the inner fountain of the realized soul rather than through the fulfillment of fleeting outer desires. Tapped into this unending reservoir of happiness, one radiates it in every direction, magnetizing people who are drawn to the light of joy and showering them with blessings. Infinite Consciousness is aware of and inherent in all things manifest and unmanifest.

Satchitananda

The *Vedas* describe Infinite Consciousness as *sat-chit-ananda*. *Sat* means "ever existing." *Chit* means "ever conscious." *Ananda* means "ever-new joy." Satchitananda encompasses all the names and images we can imagine for the One: Source of Everything, Divine Spirit, Sustainer of Life, Eternal Guiding Principle, Divine Consciousness, Inner Light, Supreme Consciousness, Divine Self, the Light Within, Supreme Self, Divine Truth, Iswara, God, the Indweller, Beloved, Infinite One, Animating Principle, Universal Consciousness, the Oneness, Ever Blissful Light Within, or Love. What we call it is not as important as full surrender to it. Only in this way is Samadhi attained.

To do this, we must release any intellectual, social, or religious concepts we have, so that we can clearly experience It from within, in meditation where It reveals Itself to us directly. We invite this revelation by humbly offering our individual ego self back to It in loving devotion.

Levels of Samadhi

To touch this state of being through the dedicated practice of the Eight Limbs is entirely within our reach and liberation is possible in this lifetime. Momentary realizations of Self that happen spontaneously during deep meditation are called Savikalpa Samadhi. Although these moments of expanded awareness are blissful, they are often unsustained and consciousness returns to its belief in separation and limitation, the resumption of "I" consciousness.

The more we practice, the more we will maintain this state of consciousness in meditation and in daily life, and the happier we will feel regardless of outer circumstances.

Eventually, the time comes for each soul when all Karma has been fully and finally released, and mastery has been attained over the transitory experience of human life. Willingness is rewarded with assurance and we lose nothing but gain everything. All masculine and feminine qualities integrate within us and we continue to operate our beautiful, individual vessels but now in complete harmony and without the perception of separateness that causes suffering. By merging individual consciousness with Divine Consciousness, we live in the world but not of it. We have entered the union that is True Yoga, where our consciousness remains forever liberated in Nirvikalpa Samadhi, or full enlightenment.

Feeling the Love

At its root, all desire is the longing of the soul to be reunited with Source. Although pain and suffering may be the initial impulses that compel us to start this journey home, only love will take us all the way. Love is the greatest motivator of all.

When we recognize all our outer strivings toward happiness as our soul's longing to be reunited with its Source, falling into love with the One is effortless. The more we relate everything back to the Divine, recognizing one love flowing through an infinite number of forms, the more we open to a greater experience of love. The ubiquitous, non-personalized love shines through all beings and we feel perpetually connected to it, intimately and at all times, not just through friends and family but throughout creation. There is no more "I" to love "you." Rather, love becomes our state of being, in which we recognize ourselves and others *as* love and the whole world as the Beloved. What we call happiness is just the tiniest little experience of that state, momentarily shining through human consciousness.

The reunion of individual consciousness with Universal Consciousness that is the goal of the Eight Limbs of Yoga is possible for all of us through diligent effort and deep devotion. No obstacle can stand in our way if we determine to succeed. Yoga is a spiritual science and the purpose of it is to prove our boundless nature. We must know personal communion with the Divine through our own consciousness. No other way will satisfy, and excuses for delay are invalid. Even tiny steps in this direction bring a substantial increase in our daily happiness levels and ability to withstand life's inevitable challenges.

Eventually an opening occurs in our hearts and minds. As the soul reawakens to its immortal nature, gaining mastery over the vehicles of body and mind rather than being limited by them, an enduring peace, coupled with an ever-increasing sense of bliss (Samadhi) are our constant companions. Life becomes a joyful game played with the abiding assurance in the unity and perfection of all creation rather than an exercise in endurance and survival. We no longer walk in fear or uncertainty for we are connected to the power that creates and sustains us. We feel a greater ease and lightness of being throughout each day and all that it brings. When trials come, we see life as a school and we rise in our consciousness to a higher, broader viewpoint.

Our practice of meditation anchors us in contact with Divine Love and enables us to give understanding, forgiveness, and goodwill to others. All of our relationships improve. We have reached the inner wellspring of happiness that everyone desires.

Only Joy

"Every saint who has penetrated to the core of reality has testified that a divine universal plan exists and that it is beautiful and full of joy," wrote Paramahansa Yogananda in *Autobiography of a Yogi.* [12]

The gift and blessing of the Yoga Sutras is that they give us clear guidance on how to follow the saints and prove this Truth. When Samadhi is entered and individual consciousness unites with Divine Consciousness, a joy is known that is millions of times more beautiful, more vast, and more enduring than any earthly pleasure we can imagine. From Joy we have come. In Joy we live, move, and have our being. And into sacred Joy we will melt again. By holding onto this, no matter what life brings, we have the key to security, freedom, perpetual happiness, and true spiritual fulfillment.

---

12   Paramahansa Yogananda, *Autobiography of a Yogi* (Los Angeles: Self Realization Fellowship, 1998), 420.

DAILY PRACTICE

Remain consistent with all of the practices of the Eight Limbs. Trust the process of spiritual evolution that they bring. Whether you touch the bliss of Samadhi momentarily or become a master of enlightenment in this lifetime, from here on it is simply joy.

QUESTIONS FOR FURTHER REFLECTION

Take a moment with your journal now to answer the following questions. Or find a quiet pause sometime today to remember the freedom and transcendence that awaits and contemplate these thoughts further.

- How can you open yourself more to the mystery of All That Is?

- If you truly knew you were an unlimited Divine being, how would this alter your daily life?

- If you recognize that your smallest actions influence the entire rest of creation, how could you be more mindful?

- How can you expand your love today?

AFFIRMATIONS TO POST AND REMEMBER

Affirmations solidify beliefs in our subconscious minds, creating a foundation from which we can then manifest positive change in our outer lives. Repeat these often with strong intensity and full faith.

- I put in my devoted effort and open to Love's grace.

- As I expand my consciousness, blessings abound.

- I am love. Love is all.

Epilogue

The end of a book is a bit like the end of a life. This unique creation had its time, took its journey, and now passes its wisdom on to the next generation. Like any life, one hopes that it holds something of lasting value to those who come after.

Last year I had the sad privilege of caring for my mother at the end of her human life. In the two weeks before her passing, I was challenged to practice every ounce of what is in this book, moment by moment, day by day.

Age and disease prevented my mother from performing even routine self-care at the end. So while changing the diaper of one who had swaddled me as a baby, I practiced reverence (Ahimsa) for her body. In the struggle to balance meeting her needs and maintaining my work and family life, I shared conflicting feelings of resentment, despair, and gratitude in truthfulness (Satya) with my husband. As I gave all that I could and humbly asked for help when I could give no more, I understood the blend of honesty and generosity (Astheya).

To save energy for caregiving, I gave up what was not essential, practicing moderation (Brahmacharya). And as I realized the magnitude of love I had been blessed with from my human mom, as well as my Divine Mother, appreciation (Aparigraha) came naturally.

When long, hot days of suffering wore into cool, silent nights of sitting in the rain together, I understood the true value of purity and simplicity (Saucha). When she could no longer move anything but her hand, yet reached out to touch mine in loving presence, I knew the meaning of contentment (Santosha).

Holding strong for her wishes even when she could not remember what she had asked of me, I felt the clarifying nature of right action (Tapas). I reached for inspiration from the sacred Sutras as I shed innumerable tears and discovered new levels of Self-reflection (Swadhaya) as emotion flooded my being. And when I surrendered the whole painful situation in loving devotion (Iswara Pranidhana) to the One that binds us in Love, I felt the assurance of what lies beyond the physical realm.

To stay strong and balanced so I could function for my family and clients, I practiced right posture (Asana). Energy control (Pranayama) was vital to manage my sorrow as I sat by her bedside watching her transition. And by employing sensory withdrawal (Pratyahara) and inner focus (Dharana), I was able to reduce the vision of suffering that surrounded me on the outside and feel her sweet essence with me on the inside. In meditation (Dhyana), I was blessed to feel the connection of our souls that transcends this human life.

Although I will not say I reached Samadhi, we shared a spectacular moment in which I witnessed what it means to have the window of consciousness opened, at least temporarily.

Mom was not a yogi and had no education in these teachings. Near the end, she struggled with her religious beliefs, feeling unable to answer the profound questions that inevitably arise near death. Even though we had spoken of spiritual topics my whole life, she became lost and confused in her beliefs.

Her time of passing was drawing near and for several days she had been mostly sleeping, barely moving or even opening her eyes. Then one day, she called to me faintly. I went to her side and held her hand. Her eyes remained closed but she was smiling. She said, "I can see now. And it is *so beautiful.*"

That was the last thing she said to me and I will never forget the peace I felt in her and in the room as she whispered those words. She had seen beyond the veil of ignorance and illusion to what is real and eternal.

There is a profound purity near death that strips away the personality that we work so hard to protect in life. The "I" really does go away and merge into what makes all of this exist. And in that mergence there is peace, and love, and bliss, just as the Eight Limbs of Yoga teach. The good news is we do not have to wait until death to experience these. They are right here, right now, available and within our reach, if we but choose them.

With every ended life, there comes a legacy. If we are lucky, that legacy is love. For Mom, it certainly is. And for this book as well, I hope. There is nothing greater than love. It is the Essence of who we all are. May joy guide your way as you practice True Yoga and may you realize your Self as Love.

—Aum, shanti, shanti, shanti, Aum.

Jennie Lee

Recommended Resources

Bouanchaud, Bernard. *The Essence of Yoga: Reflections on the Yoga Sutras of Patanjali.* Delhi: Indian Books Centre, 1997.

Cope, Stephen. *Yoga & the Quest for the True Self.* New York: Bantam, 2000.

Desikachar, T.K.V. *The Heart of Yoga: Developing a Personal Practice.* Rochester, VT: Inner Traditions International, 1995.

Devi, Nischala Joy. *The Secret Power of Yoga: A Woman's Guide to the Heart and Spirit of the Yoga Sutras.* New York: Three Rivers Press, 2007.

Dyer, Wayne. *There's a Spiritual Solution to Every Problem.* New York: Harper Collins, 2001.

Easwaran, Eknath. *Gandhi the Man: The Story of His Transformation.* Berkeley: Nilgiri Press, 1997.

———. *The Upanishads.* Berkeley: Nilgiri Press, 1987.

Farhi, Donna. *Bringing Yoga to Life: The Everyday Practice of Enlightened Living.* New York: Harper Collins, 2005.

Feuerstein, Georg. *The Yoga Tradition: Its History, Literature, Philosophy and Practice.* Chino Valley, AZ: Hohm Press, 2001.

Gandhi, M. K. *The Way to God.* Berkeley: Berkeley Hills Books, 1999.

Judith, Anodea. *Wheels of Life: A User's Guide to the Chakra System.* Woodbury, MN: Llewellyn Worldwide, 1987.

Kraftsow, Gary. *Yoga for Transformation: Ancient Teachings and Practices for Healing the Body, Mind and Heart.* New York: Penguin Books, 2002.

Lasater, Judith Hanson. *Living Your Yoga: Finding the Spiritual in Everyday Life.* Berkeley: Rodmell Press, 1999.

Levine, Stephen. *The Gradual Awakening.* New York: Anchor Press, 1989.

Satchidananda, Sri Swami. *The Yoga Sutras of Patanjali.* Buckingham, VA: Integral Yoga Publications, 2012.

Singer, Michael. *The Untethered Soul: The Journey Beyond Yourself.* Oakland, CA: New Harbinger, 2007.

Sivananda Radha, Swami. *Hatha Yoga: The Hidden Language, Symbols, Secrets and Metaphors.* Canada: Timeless Books, 2006.

Weintraub, Amy. *Yoga for Depression: A Compassionate Guide to Relieve Suffering Through Yoga.* New York: Broadway Books, 2004.

Williamson, Marianne. *A Return to Love: Reflections on the Principles of "A Course in Miracles."* San Francisco: Harper One, 1996.

Yogananda, Paramahansa. *Autobiography of a Yogi.* Los Angeles: Self Realization Fellowship, 1998.

———. *The Divine Romance: Collected Talks and Essays on Realizing God in Daily Life, Volume II.* Los Angeles: Self Realization Fellowship, 2005.

———. *The Yoga of the Bhagavad Gita.* Los Angeles: Self Realization Fellowship, 2008.

Yukteswar Giri, Sri Swami. *The Holy Science.* Dakshineswar: Yogoda Satsanga Society of India, 1990.

Index

Acknowledgments

I hold deepest gratitude and love for the following people, without whom this book would not be.

- My husband Larry for his unfailing love and support.

- My son Benen for making me laugh and challenging me to live my yoga more every day.

- My guru Paramahansa Yogananda for his inspiration and loving assurance.

- My mom Jeanne for always believing in me.

- My friend Michael for helping me expand my understanding of God.

- My daughter Carina Rose for rebirthing the spiritual warrior in me.

- My friend Dave for relentlessly educating people on what true yoga is.

- My meditation sanghas on O'ahu for their consistent embrace.

- My friend Bridget for holding my hand at the beginning of the journey.

- My agent Steve for never giving up.

- My editor Angela for believing in my vision and for working so very hard to manifest it.

- My team at Llewellyn Worldwide for all their hard work and support.